1-02

W9-CDT-955

THE
FIBROMYALGIA
HANDBOOK

HARRIS H. McILWAIN, M.D.
DEBRA FULGHUM BRUCE

Second Edition
REVISED AND EXPANDED

AN OWL BOOK
HENRY HOLT AND COMPANY
NEW YORK

Henry Holt and Company, LLC
Publishers since 1866
115 West 18th Street
New York, New York 10011

Henry Holt® is a registered trademark
of Henry Holt and Company, LLC.

Published in Canada by Fitzhenry & Whiteside Ltd.,
195 Allstate Parkway, Markham, Ontario L3R 4T8.

Library of Congress Cataloging-in-Publication Data
McIlwain, Harris H.
    The fibromyalgia handbook / Harris H. McIlwain
    and Debra Fulghum Bruce.
    p.   cm.
    Includes bibliographical references and index.
    ISBN 0-8050-6115-0
    1. Fibromyalgia—Handbooks, manuals, etc.
    I. Bruce, Debra Fulghum.   II. Title.
    RC927.3M36   1996   96-16846
    616.7'4—dc20   CIP

Henry Holt books are available for special promotions and
premiums. For details contact: Director, Special Markets.

Second Edition 1999

Designed by Ann Gold

Printed in the United States of America

10   9   8   7   6   5

This book is not intended as a substitute for medical advice of physicians and should
be used only in conjunction with the advice of your personal doctor. The reader should
regularly consult a physician in matters relating to his or her health and particularly
with respect to any symptoms that may require diagnosis or medical attention.

CONTENTS

THE FIBROMYALGIA HANDBOOK

INTRODUCTION: YOU HAVEN'T GOT TIME FOR THE PAIN

If you have been diagnosed with fibromyalgia, fibrositis, or myofascial pain syndrome, no one needs to tell you of the almost daily muscle pain you live with, along with constant fatigue, sleeplessness, and low-grade depression. As a rheumatologist for more than twenty years, I have seen fibromyalgia take its toll on once healthy individuals, mostly women ages twenty to sixty. Not only does it strike during young and middle adult years, the busiest and most stressful time of one's life, but patients tell of the symptoms making them feel as if they are 100 years old. The good news is that *it does not have to be this way!* You can live actively with fibromyalgia, *if* you learn how to manage its symptoms.

Years ago, it became apparent to doctors that patients who told of having muscle aches, fatigue, depression, headaches, and sleeplessness were harboring a distinct disease or syndrome (a collection of symptoms that make a disease). Yet the results from lab tests and X rays were always normal. Two decades ago, physicians sent these patients home with few answers, as we could only treat the symptoms.

Today we know differently. In the past five years there has been a plethora of research done on this mysterious syndrome we call "fibromyalgia" or FMS. Now millions of people can understand that the disease is real; the symptoms are *not* imagined *nor* did they cause them; and treatment does work, if followed faithfully.

A View of Fibromyalgia

In this book, you will become knowledgeable about fibromyalgia and learn how to lessen the severity of the symptoms. Questions will be addressed, such as:

- Does being overweight make one more likely to get fibromyalgia?
- Why is this considered a "female" disease?
- Does estrogen have anything to do with it?
- Is there a cure for this or will it continue to cause pain for my entire life?
- Should I push myself on days when the pain and fatigue seem unbearable?
- How do I know which medications will help me?
- How can I know for sure that this is fibromyalgia?
- Will the disease run its course?
- Did I cause the disease from too much stress or poor nutrition?
- Does exercise hurt or help the painful symptoms?
- Is it inherited?

While there are no cures for fibromyalgia, you can learn to control your specific symptoms as you manage the disease with the 7-Step Treatment Program. This plan has proved to be successful with thousands of my patients as they identify the symptoms of the disease, carefully seek a diagnosis, and learn to manage the disease in a reasonable way.

Let's look at some patients who have taken the steps needed to control their fibromyalgia and are winning with this disease.

Chronic Fatigue and Muscle Pain

Linda was one patient who benefited greatly from the combination 7-Step Treatment Program outlined in this book. After her youngest child entered elementary school, this thirty-nine-year-old woman enrolled at the local university to work on her master's degree. Halfway through the quarter, Linda noticed a dramatic change in her health. "I've always needed eight hours of sleep," she said upon evaluation. "But for the past month, I have been sleeping eleven or twelve hours and still feel tired when I awaken."

This once active woman told of feeling so chronically fatigued that even walking to class from a nearby parking lot left her feeling weak. She said that even a cool breeze on her skin felt like burning fire and the only relief she could get from this pain was lying down in bed. "Imagine feeling like you had worked out for hours, yet all you did was make your breakfast and take a shower."

After seeing three physicians, including a sleep disorders specialist who ruled out any nighttime respiratory problems, Linda came to our clinic. In the meantime, Linda continued to take courses while maintaining a family. But the added stress of going to school and studying took its toll, for she felt overwrought, as if her body was failing her.

Upon diagnosis, Linda began the 7-Step Treatment Program, including a specific focus on dietary changes (see chapter 8), stress reduction, and gentle stretching exercises several times a day. As predicted, her symptoms responded positively. Within three weeks, Linda felt relief from the constant, nagging pain and was able to increase her normal activity.

Hot, Searing Leg Pain

Jean, a high school principal, told of being unable to walk one morning about five years ago. "I'll never forget that day for as long as I live. I had set my alarm early that morning because the accreditation team was coming to the school for our annual review.

"When I put my feet on the floor, my legs simply gave way. My left ankle had a hot, searing, and burning pain that went throughout the heel, arch, and toes. When I sat on my right hip, my thigh and leg hurt so badly, it was unbearable. There was a pinching feeling in my hip and I could hardly walk. All I could think of was that my career was over."

After a CT (computerized tomography) scan and MRI (magnetic resonance imaging)—two commonly used imaging techniques to see inside the body—showed no medical reason for her pain, Jean came to our clinic for an evaluation. She had been told by two doctors that her pain was a mental health problem, yet as an educator, she knew there was more to it. In fact, her symptoms of pain and fatigue were so relentless that it took several months to get this under control.

As Linda and thousands have experienced, once Jean received the diagnosis of fibromyalgia and began the treatment program, she was able to increase activity and live a normal life again.

Achiness, Fatigue, and Depression

When Elizabeth, a forty-five-year-old attorney, got over a recent bout with the flu, she thought that the achiness that lingered was from being run down. "I had this unending pain that made me so depressed. I even thought that death would be a welcome relief, because I hurt all over. The pain became so intense that I couldn't have sex with my husband without tears, yet he did not seem to understand. I couldn't even do light household chores without wanting to scream out in agony."

It took three months of doctors' appointments until Elizabeth's symptoms were finally given a name—fibromyalgia.

"How could doctors look me straight in the eye and say that the pain and fatigue were in my head? One doctor said that a cruise would make me feel less stressed. A cruise? I didn't need a cruise, I needed a diagnosis, and, more importantly, I needed a form of treatment."

For Elizabeth, living with fibromyalgia has been an eye-opening experience. "It is hard to realize that healthy people can get this disease, but they can. I now understand that education is the key in controlling the symptoms."

Most important, the quality of life for Linda, Jean, and Elizabeth has greatly improved since starting the treatment plan. All three tell of now sleeping soundly, having more energy, and feeling less pressure since they took control of the debilitating symptoms.

From Patient to Person

What is the goal of living with this disease? You should strive to change the disease from something disabling to something manageable. With the 7-Step Treatment Program, you can learn to treat each symptom in a positive manner, doing the activities you enjoy in reasonable comfort without being overly medicated or feeling debilitating pain and stiffness.

You deserve to know that the high anxiety that accompanies fibromyalgia can make you feel broken, especially when you haven't got time for the pain, fatigue, and immobility. However, in the midst of the brokenness that you feel, I know that you can become a *whole person* again as you learn to conquer this disease instead of conceding to it.

Now let's get started.

1

WHAT IS
FIBROMYALGIA?

A ching, stabbing, and sometimes even pulsating." That's how forty-one-year-old Kelly, an FMS survivor, described the unending deep muscle pain in her neck, shoulders, and knees. "The pain stays with me from the moment I get up until I literally crawl into bed at night.

"I feel pain most when I have to keep up with my three children, driving carpools, cooking dinners, or making sure everyone has clothes ironed for school the next day. But, honestly, there are increasingly more days when I can hardly take care of my own needs, much less my children's needs, because of sheer exhaustion from the interminable pain."

Aren't there times when you can identify with Kelly? We all get tired. And who doesn't feel sore, achy, and stiff, especially after a weekend of sports activities or heavy gardening? Yet for those like Kelly with FMS, these symptoms are chronic and severe. The debilitating symptoms of never-ending muscle pain and fatigue are constant, lasting for months and years and causing poor quality of life for its millions of victims—damaging jobs, families, and personal lives.

Rebecca came to our clinic because of widespread pain that she described as "stabbing and throbbing" from her shoulders and the back of her neck to her legs. This forty-seven-year-old woman worked full-time as a data processor, but in the past few months she had been unable to sit at the computer for any length of time due to the pain.

"I wake up every day with stabbing pain and think that maybe it will go away," she said. "When I get to work and sit at the computer, the pain worsens and often feels piercing, like a knife is in my muscle. I feel tired all the time and can't cook dinner for my family. If anyone touches me, I cringe because of the tenderness. Because of the exhaustion, I'm in bed by 7:30 P.M. each night, yet I never feel rested. What is wrong with me?"

After a careful examination and evaluation of the symptoms, this middle-aged woman was diagnosed with fibromyalgia. Coined in 1976, the term *fibromyalgia* describes the basic symptoms of constant muscle pain, tenderness, fatigue, and tender points. As Rebecca experienced, fibromyalgia causes widespread pain—in the back, neck, arms, and legs— with many tender or trigger points that are very painful when touched.

Fibromyalgia—with its deep muscle pain, disturbed sleep, and feelings of depression—affects more than 10 million Americans, with 90 percent or more being women aged forty to fifty or older. There are new estimates that as many as 8 percent of *all* women are affected by fibromyalgia. This may bring some comfort to the millions of women who thought the symptoms of fatigue, aching muscles, and low-grade depression were "mental" in nature.

Sophisticated research has shown that the syndrome can start in childhood or teenage years, especially with girls, and gradually worsens with age. Some recent studies show that because of the common symptoms, the disease may be vastly underdiagnosed in older adults, who often accept the unexplained pain in their bodies as another sign of aging. It is important to know up front that fibromyalgia is *not* a sign of aging!

Patients tell of going from doctor to doctor with symptoms of fatigue, which are present even on arising. They may have specific *tender points* on the body that hurt to the touch, or they may have pain all over. Forty-one-year-old Janis told of hurting everywhere on her body; even sitting in a straight-back chair brought tears to her eyes. Sarah, a young mother of two, felt throbbing pain all over her body as well as disturbances in deep-level, restful sleep, accompanied by sadness or depression. Mike felt a piercing pain in his neck and shoulders, accompanied by sluggishness, that came on suddenly after a car accident. While these patients had different manifestations of pain and fatigue, the symptoms were all the result of fibromyalgia.

A Common but Misunderstood Disease

Even though this has been a commonly misdiagnosed and misunderstood syndrome, fibromyalgia is the most common arthritis-related disease next to osteoarthritis. The consensus document on fibromyalgia from the Second World Conference on Myofascial Pain and Fibromyalgia in 1992 reported that fibromyalgia may be the most common cause of widespread musculoskeletal pain.

Fibromyalgia was first described in medical documents more than 150 years ago, yet even as recent as ten years ago, this problem was rarely discussed in the medical community. Those who don't understand it may not recognize that it exists. One middle-aged woman recently brought her entire family into our clinic to talk about FMS. "Because I look healthy, they think I overexaggerate my symptoms," she explained. "Please tell them that I'm not making this up."

One must wonder how treatment can begin if the problem is not recognized. For most people, it is common for the symptoms to drag on for months or years before a proper diagnosis is made. In fact, for most patients, the average amount of time to pass before diagnosis is made is *four to five years*. Imagine living half a decade with debilitating symptoms and being told by family, friends, and your physician that the pain and fatigue are in your head!

Thousands of patients each year tell of going from doctor to doctor with symptoms of crippling fatigue and constant muscle and joint pain all over their body. "Before I was diagnosed with fibromyalgia, I was told by two doctors that nothing was wrong with me," Vicky said, "and another suggested that my pain was psychological."

While more and more people are receiving the proper diagnosis of fibromyalgia from physicians who understand this rheumatic disease, there are estimates that thousands of people are still living with undiagnosed and untreated symptoms.

If you have been diagnosed with fibromyalgia or if you have the described symptoms and believe that this might be the problem, you have probably heard one or more of the following statements from friends and family members:

"It's all in your head."

"If you would relax more, you could sleep at night."

"Maybe you're too focused on yourself; get out and get busy."

"If you would exercise more, you wouldn't feel that muscle pain."

"Get a job. It will make you feel less depressed."

"You look healthy to me. Maybe you just want sympathy."

"You just don't want to feel good. Why do you always crave attention?"

"Slow down. Your life is so busy, it is making you crazy."

"Your life is wonderful, so don't be depressed."

"If the doctor says it's in your head, it must be true."

"If the lab tests do not show anything, you aren't sick."

"You act like this is the end of the world; lighten up."

After suffering with endless pain and chronic fatigue day after day, month after month, you may even begin to believe that you are fabricating the symptoms or that the problem really is in your mind. But this disease is very real.

Lydia, a forty-two-year-old lab technician and mother of two, was faced with early retirement due to the fatigue and even had to take catnaps throughout her workday to keep going. Lydia told of feeling widespread aching and stabbing pain in her muscles and joints, which greatly affected her ability to work and care for her family. She lived with these symptoms for four years and was evaluated by six doctors but did not receive a correct diagnosis.

When she came to our clinic, she felt tired, achy, and mildly depressed. But more important, Lydia was angry that no one could tell her what was happening to her body. "I guess because my symptoms and feelings come and go, the doctors thought that I was overworked or depressed," she said. "The antidepressant one doctor prescribed helped me sleep, but I still didn't feel rested in the morning, and I continued to hurt all over."

Darlene came to our clinic complaining of searing pain in her back, neck, and chest, along with throbbing headaches that occurred almost daily. This forty-five-year-old legal secretary and single mother of three had very specific *tender points* on the body that were painful to touch, along with regular disturbances in deep-level or restful sleep at night. Her main concern was the stiffness throughout her body on arising in the morning. "I have to work, but after walking up the stairs to my office, the pain is unbearable," she said.

Darlene's excruciating pain was worsened by any stress, a symptom that is quite common. She said that when the disease was active, her concentration at work was gravely affected, and she felt more irritable, even depressed. Another patient, forty-year-old Nina, had deep muscle pain in the abdomen along with dramatic changes in her bowel habits, ranging from constipation to diarrhea.

Darlene and Nina had frequency in urination with a sensation of an immediate urge to urinate; and both women complained of painful menstrual cramps, which are quite common in women with fibromyalgia. Nina had a pale discoloration of the fingers on cold exposure, such as holding a cold glass or putting a hand in the refrigerator.

Sick or Old?

Peter, a middle-aged gentleman, came to see me about his symptoms, which had been ongoing for several months. He seemed a bit nervous during our conversation, then admitted that on the day of his evaluation, he was symptom-free. "I don't understand it," Peter said. "The last few days, I didn't ache at all, and last night I slept for the first time without tossing and turning."

Peter's case is not unusual. In fibromyalgia, the symptoms may come and go; therefore, it may be difficult to get proper diagnosis. If the physician does not understand the complexity of the disease, a patient may be sent away without any help or hope for treatment. In fact, studies show that *thousands* of patients each year tell of going from doctor to doctor with constant pain all over their body along with feelings of fatigue. Many are told that there is nothing wrong or that the problem is psychological.

Today we know differently. We know that fibromyalgia is a complex disorder characterized by *chronic* (meaning three months or longer) widespread pain, decreased pain threshold or tender points, and incapacitating fatigue. Women are ten times more likely to get the disease than men. While there is no specific laboratory test or abnormal X ray finding for diagnosis, the symptoms of the disease can be successfully treated once a proper diagnosis is made.

The Causes of Fibromyalgia

HYPERSENSITIVE TO PAIN?

Through numerous clinical studies, researchers have found that in people who suffer with chronic pain, the spinal cord becomes overloaded with input. This may make it oversensitive to any messages sent its way and causes the spinal cord to overreact to or amplify any response. When your body reacts hypersensitively in this way to pain, even a gentle breeze touching your skin will make you hurt. Recently scientists have concluded that fibromyalgia patients often feel higher sensitivity to pain over their entire body. This has led to the idea that with FMS, the body's overall pain threshold may be dramatically lower than usual.

Some researchers think fibromyalgia may be the result of a genetic tendency; therefore, it may be passed on from generation to generation. When a person who has this tendency is exposed to certain emotional or physical stressors (like an illness or life crisis), there is a change in the body's response to stress. This can result in a higher sensitivity of the entire body to pain. Scientists theorize that one of these body changes is a low level of a hormone, CRH (corticotropin-releasing hormone), resulting in higher sensitivity to pain and more fatigue, including the fatigue experienced after exercise. Still other researchers have recently concluded that those with fibromyalgia have significantly less blood flow to the parts of the brain that deal with pain. In studies where fibromyalgia patients were compared to healthy people, those with FMS were found to have twice the level of a brain chemical called *substance P,* a neuropeptide involved in pain signals. This chemical helps nervous system cells send messages to each other about painful stimuli. It is thought that when P levels are elevated in the body, they may produce higher levels of pain.

LINKED TO STRESS OR TRAUMA TO NERVOUS SYSTEM?

Researchers indicate that fibromyalgia is linked to stress or emotional illness. On the other hand, some studies show that psychological stress in the patient is often high *before* the disease begins. Although it is not known why, researchers are finding that fibromyalgia may be caused by biochemical changes in the body, for example, accidents, injuries, or illnesses. Other studies reveal that the disease may result from sudden trauma to the central nervous system.

A RESULT OF MENOPAUSE?

"Since I went into menopause, my symptoms have quadrupled," Lois, a fifty-four-year-old retired teacher who was diagnosed three years ago, said. "I had to quit teaching kindergarten because the pain in my shoulders and neck kept me from keeping up with my kids, and I felt so tired each day."

Some researchers have suggested that the loss of the female hormone *estrogen,* which happens at menopause, may trigger this disease. Hosts of experiments are being done to see if loss of estrogen does, in fact, stimulate this disease; it is true that fibromyalgia occurs more commonly between the ages of forty to fifty-five, or around the time of menopause.

DUE TO AGING?

"Maybe fibromyalgia is similar to aging," Nancy surmised. "All these symptoms came on at midlife, and I have heard that all things fall apart after age forty."

The truth is that even though the disease occurs more frequently after the age of forty, there is no specific evidence that fibromyalgia is a problem of aging. It is also well known to occur in teenagers and gradually worsen over time. It does not continue to increase in much older people (seventy to eighty years old).

CONNECTED TO SEROTONIN?

Clearly, some research indicates that other possible causes could be a deficiency of one of the body's chemicals, *serotonin,* or its precursor, *tryptophan,* or even *magnesium.* Serotonin is a neurotransmitter in the brain associated with a calming, anxiety-reducing reaction. Lower levels of serotonin cause a lower pain threshold. The end result may be the chronic widespread pain of fibromyalgia. These findings may also explain the sleep problems associated with this disease.

AFTER INJURY OR AS A RESULT OF LYME DISEASE?

Fibromyalgia often occurs following an injury, even one that may be mild, or after a bout with the flu. Some patients diagnosed with Lyme disease, which can cause muscle and joint pain, along with other problems, and is spread through the bite of a tick, were found to have fibromyalgia as their main problem. No specific evidence was found that Lyme disease caused fibromyalgia in those patients.

POOR PHYSICAL CONDITIONING OR AS A RESULT OF DEPRESSION?

Some studies support the theory that people who are unfit are more likely to get fibromyalgia. Speculation is that stress and poor physical conditioning may both be major factors in the cause of the disease.

Other studies have shown that because fibromyalgia is accompanied by low-grade depression, there may be a link between these two illnesses. Some researchers feel that depression leads to changes in the chemistry of the brain or that abnormalities of the sympathetic nervous system result in the release of substances that cause more sensitivity to pain, resulting in fibromyalgia.

UNKNOWN CAUSES?

Although there are many theories on what causes fibromyalgia, the truth remains unknown. For many years doctors thought that the disease was caused by a disorder of the muscles or that it was a psychological problem. Some researchers believe that this mysterious syndrome has a genetic disposition, as it can run in families. The most recent research suggests that the muscles themselves are not the source of the pain, but rather that the pain is a response to changes in the brain. All of these explanations remain unproven, but research is continuing.

No single theory seems to explain all of the problems in fibromyalgia. Whatever the cause, the vicious cycle of pain and disturbed sleep leads to less activity, greater depression, and more pain. This pain cycle can incapacitate the sufferer for months and possibly years unless the proper treatment is administered to control the symptoms. While there is no cure, the symptoms *can* be successfully treated.

Fibromyalgia and Other Illnesses

If what current research indicates is true, other factors play a role in increasing or lessening fibromyalgia's symptoms. We know that when other illnesses or diseases are present, symptoms can greatly accelerate, causing more pain, fatigue, and anxiety or depression. FMS can worsen during times of great stress or after exercise. Conversely, the chronic pain can subside during less stressful times. Beverly, age thirty-seven, told of living with chronic pain for months. Then, during a two-week cruise to the Caribbean with her husband, she became almost pain-free.

"After a few days into the cruise, I started sleeping through the night without awakening, and I was able to sightsee without resting periodically for the muscle pain. I thought I was healed, except that it was short-lived.

"Almost one month after my vacation, the pain started again, and it was worse than ever. Somehow, I know that lessening my stress helped me reduce symptoms."

FIBROMYALGIA CLASSIFICATIONS

1. Fibromyalgia without any other underlying disease, such as osteoarthritis or other types of arthritis.
2. Fibromyalgia along with another disease, such as osteoarthritis, rheumatoid arthritis, or systemic lupus erythematosus (SLE).

The Feelings of Fibromyalgia

Because fibromyalgia can cause signs and feelings similar to osteoarthritis, bursitis, and tendinitis, some specialists include it in the group of arthritis and related disorders. But unlike the bursitis or tendinitis, which is usually localized to a single area, the feelings of pain and stiffness associated with fibromyalgia are widespread. In fact, if there are not many areas involved, then it does not fit the typical picture of fibromyalgia. If a joint is warm or swollen or does not move properly, then there is probably another problem present, such as another form of arthritis or an injury.

For some patients, fibromyalgia's symptoms are not always constant—the pain comes and goes. Unlike some severe forms of arthritis that cause crippling, most fibromyalgia patients are able to get through the day, though they constantly feel tired and achy.

COMMON SYMPTOMS OF FIBROMYALGIA

Pain
Fatigue
Morning stiffness
Trigger points
Sleep problems
Anxiety
Difficulty in concentration
Depression

Swelling, numbness, and tingling in hands, arms, feet,
  and legs
Headaches
Irritable bowel syndrome (abdominal pain, constipation,
  diarrhea)
Urinary symptoms (burning, frequency)
Painful menstrual cramps
Discoloration of hands and feet (Raynaud's phenomenon)
Restless legs syndrome
Dryness in mouth, nose, and eyes

PAIN: THE MOST COMMON SYMPTOM

Pain plays a significant role in the diagnosis of fibromyalgia
and is usually the major complaint that signals a visit to the
doctor. This widespread pain is characteristic of more than 97
percent of patients. Unlike the pain of osteoarthritis, bursitis,
or tendinitis, which is usually relegated to a specific joint or
area, this pain can be felt over the entire body and is deep,
sharp, dull, throbbing, or aching. There may also be accompanying pain in the joints, such as the shoulders, hips, back, and
neck. Joint pain can also come from the hands, wrists, elbows,
knees, ankles, and feet. However, even more common is pain
felt in the muscles, tendons, and ligaments around the joints.

Peggy was diagnosed strictly from the pain she was experiencing. "I live day and night with a sharp, throbbing pain in the
muscles in my neck and shoulders, yet I have not experienced
the fatigue that usually accompanies this. The pain becomes
especially intense after exercise or housework, especially when
I do such chores as sweeping, mopping, vacuuming, or washing
windows. The pain becomes so unbearable that sometimes prescription pain medications do not touch it."

Other patients who tell of feeling pain in the back, neck,
and head complain also of frequent headaches. Many times
these pains are from the muscles and other soft tissues around
the back and neck, not from fibromyalgia.

I often see patients who have had a back injury, such as a

ruptured disc in the lower part of the spine (lumbar spine). These patients have had surgery on the lower back or neck for treatment of the injury. After a back injury, which may result in bed rest and loss of activity, many patients develop symptoms of fibromyalgia for reasons that are unknown.

RELENTLESS FATIGUE IS CRIPPLING

Next to pain and the tender trigger points, fatigue is a major complaint. We *all* know what it feels like to be tired. However, because we are each different, we may have dissimilar ideas of the meaning of *fatigue*. What is fatigue to you may not be the same for me or someone else. Fatigue in fibromyalgia refers to a lingering tiredness that is constant and limiting. For example, patients complain of being tired even when they should feel rested and have had enough sleep. Some patients admit to feeling sleepy, but much more common is a feeling of exhaustion without feeling drowsy. Some compare it to having the flu or to the feeling after working very long hours and missing a lot of sleep.

Just as the cause of fibromyalgia is not known, the exact cause of the fatigue is not known. Sleep disturbances, common in the large majority of patients, may help create a constant state of fatigue. In fact, hosts of experiments have shown that many of fibromyalgia's symptoms can actually be created in otherwise healthy people if their sleep is disturbed. Fatigue is so bothersome in many patients that they often say, "Please get rid of the fatigue, and I'll put up with the pain."

THE FATIGUE OF FIBROMYALGIA

Fatigued on arising in the morning

Fatigued after mild activity, such as grocery shopping or cooking dinner

Too fatigued to start a project, such as folding clothes or ironing

Too fatigued to exercise

Even more fatigued after exercise

Too fatigued for sex
Too fatigued to function adequately at work

MORNING STIFFNESS AFFECTS MOST PATIENTS

More than 75 percent of fibromyalgia patients feel stiffness in
the morning on arising. This stiffness creates a feeling of the
need to loosen up after getting out of bed before usual activities can begin, and the stiffness is extensive, going throughout
the muscles and joints of the back, arms, and legs. In some
patients, the morning stiffness may last only a few minutes,
but it is usually very noticeable for more than fifteen or twenty
minutes each day. Other patients report that the stiffness lasts
for hours or even seems to be present all day. Most people
feel stiff when they wake up, but this type of stiffness is very
different than minor aching. In fact, this is the same feeling of
stiffness in the morning that happens in many types of arthritis, especially rheumatoid arthritis.

TRIGGER POINTS

Many influences are at work in fibromyalgia. Patients like
Peggy feel sharp, throbbing muscle pain. But accompanying
this deep muscle soreness are painful *trigger points,* or localized areas of tenderness around joints (not joints themselves)
that hurt when pressed with a finger. These can be deep areas
of pain but are often superficial areas seemingly under the
surface of the skin, such as over the elbow or shoulder.

The cause of these trigger points is not known. Even
though it would seem that these areas should be inflamed, no
particular signs of inflammation have been found by researchers when the tissues are examined. The locations of the trigger
points are not random; they are in predictable places on the
body (see page 37).

SLEEP PROBLEMS

Most people with FMS are really bothered by sleep problems.
The most common complaint is simply not having restful

sleep, which is usually related to frequent "awakenings." During these awakenings, you may not notice being fully awake, but you are aroused enough to feel unrefreshed the next morning. While some researchers hold strongly to the belief that FMS may be due to nonrestorative deep sleep, sleep disorder is not thought to be the only cause of fibromyalgia.

The exact cause of the sleep disorder is not known, but scientists have discovered abnormal amounts of *alpha activity* on an electroencephalogram taken of FMS patients. (The electroencephalogram is a test done during a sleep study or polysomnography, which is discussed in chapter 5.) Alpha activity in the brain is associated with feelings of serenity and calmness, whereas beta activity is related to alertness.

Even though poor sleep doesn't create the fibromyalgia, it can make you feel exhausted upon awakening. This results in more pain, more sleep problems, and more fatigue. Interestingly, FMS-like symptoms have been induced in normal volunteers who were deprived of sleep—except in those who regularly exercised. The reason for this is that exercise increases the time you spend in deep sleep and has been found to be an excellent therapy for FMS patients. Some ways you can begin an exercise program are discussed in chapter 4.

Some people may have coexisting sleep disorders such as restless legs syndrome or obstructive sleep apnea in addition to fibromyalgia. With restless legs syndrome, you feel a creeping, crawling sensation in the legs (and sometimes in the arms) that creates an irresistible urge to move.

Sleep apnea is a potentially life-threatening problem where a person stops breathing due to relaxed or excessive tissue blocking the airway. In these cases, going to a sleep disorder clinic for polysomnography can help in making the diagnosis and treating the symptoms.

COMMON SLEEP-RELATED SYMPTOMS WITH FMS

- I have frequent headaches in the morning upon getting out of bed.
- I feel muscle aches and pains throughout my body most of the time.
- I feel fatigue or tiredness that does not go away even after several large cups of strongly caffeinated coffee.
- I feel in a low mood that does not lift even as I get on with my daily activities.
- I have felt depressed enough to get antidepressants from my doctor.
- I feel irritable, impatient, and have mood swings.
- I often have difficulty being with a large group, as it feels overwhelming.
- I have trouble learning new information or grasping new ideas.
- I am unable to recall useful information and feel "foggy" sometimes.

DEPRESSION INTERFERES WITH ACTIVITIES

Depression and concentration problems are key symptoms with most patients. In fact, anxiety and depression severe enough to interfere with daily activities occur in 50 percent or more of fibromyalgia patients. Stress from the constant pain and fatigue can cause anxiety. The chronic pain can result in less activity, leading the patient to become more withdrawn, all of which can lead to depression.

No matter which case is eventually found to be correct, anxiety and depression can greatly interfere with a patient's activities at work and at home. The symptoms can be successfully treated with a combination of medication and therapy, so it is important to discuss these feelings openly with your doctor.

People tell of great difficulty keeping their attention concentrated on their work or other activity. Some complain of their short-term memory worsening. Although memory blanks are a common complaint, difficulty concentrating (what many call "fibro fog"), anxiety, and panic attacks are all commonly reported symptoms, too. For some people, being in a "fibro fog" may be the main complaint and limitation.

SWELLING AND TINGLING HANDS CAN BE A PROBLEM

While the cause is not known, many patients have a feeling of swelling in the hands, arms, feet, or legs. The feeling may be especially bothersome upon arising, especially in combination with morning stiffness, yet does not appear to limit activity.

Numbness or tingling sensations in the hands, arms, or legs are also reported by more than half of all fibromyalgia patients. The medical term for these feelings is *paresthesia*. The sensations happen irregularly and usually last a few minutes, though they can be constant. Although these sensations may be bothersome, they are not severely limiting.

CHRONIC HEADACHES ARE PART OF THE DISEASE

More than half of all fibromyalgia patients suffer from chronic headaches. They are often caused by tightness in and contraction of the muscles of the neck and are called *tension-type headaches* or *muscle-contraction headaches*. They may also be caused by tenderness from trigger points over the back of the head and the neck. It is important to remember that headaches can be caused by other medical problems, which should be properly diagnosed and treated by your doctor.

IRRITABLE BOWEL SYNDROME AFFECTS SUFFERERS

Irritable bowel syndrome (IBS) is a condition characterized by abdominal cramps and pain, along with periods of diarrhea alternating with bouts of constipation. About one-third of fibromyalgia patients suffer from IBS. Complaints can include excessive gas and bloating along with the irritable bowel syndrome.

URINARY FREQUENCY CAN OCCUR

A feeling of the urge to urinate, which is a condition called *urinary urgency,* painful or frequent urination, and incontinence have been found in about 25 percent of fibromyalgia patients. Since these problems can also be caused by other bladder and kidney diseases, it is important to check with your doctor to be sure no other specific problems are present.

PAINFUL MENSTRUAL CRAMPS AFFECT FEMALE PATIENTS

Unusually painful menstrual cramps are found in 30 to 40 percent of women with fibromyalgia. There are specific problems that can cause menstrual cramps, so be sure to check with your doctor to be sure no other treatment is needed.

DISCOLORATION OF EXTREMITIES

Some patients notice that their fingers or, though less commonly, their toes become pale, cold, or turn blue when exposed to cold—even such a small exposure as holding a cold glass. The pale or blue changes may last for a few minutes and can be accompanied by pain. When the hands or feet are warmed, they return to normal.

This problem is called *Raynaud's phenomenon.* It can happen in otherwise normal persons and is also a characteristic of other medical problems, such as other types of arthritis. Again, your doctor can make sure no other medical problems are present. Sometimes, medications are needed to control this symptom.

RESTLESS LEGS SYNDROME

Restless legs syndrome is a condition many fibromyalgia sufferers complain of. This is characterized by discomfort of the legs, especially below the knee, and is especially bothersome at night. The feeling can be painful and is most commonly described as the need to move the legs to try to make them comfortable. Restless legs syndrome often interrupts sleep as the sufferer tries to find the most comfortable position for rest. As with other symptoms, restless legs syndrome can be found with other medical problems and has no good treatment.

DRYNESS IS A CONCERN

Dryness of the mouth, nose, or eyes can happen in otherwise normal persons, but more than 25 percent of fibromyalgia patients have this symptom. Dryness occurs when glands do not produce the normal amounts or quality of tears to lubricate the eyes or saliva to lubricate the mouth. This problem is commonly associated with rheumatoid and other types of arthritis and is called *Sjögren's syndrome*. There is no single known cause.

Although dryness is mainly uncomfortable, the loss of normal lubrication for the eyes can increase the risk of infection. The loss of normal saliva and lubrication in the mouth increases the chance of tooth decay. See your ophthalmologist and/or dentist for treatment.

Factors That Worsen Symptoms

In many studies, patients report that weather changes greatly affect musculoskeletal symptoms. In fact, those with the highest weather sensitivity tend to have more functional impairment and psychological distress.

FACTORS THAT CAN WORSEN FIBROMYALGIA SYMPTOMS
Anxiety and depression
Changes in weather (cold or humidity)
Fatigue
Injuries
Lack of sleep or restless sleep
Other illnesses
Periods of emotional stress

Physical exhaustion
Sedentary lifestyle (lack of exercise)

Fibromyalgia with Other Diseases

Fibromyalgia can occur alone or it can occur with one of the other 100 types of arthritis. For example, you may have osteo-arthritis in the knee from an old football injury; yet you can have fibromyalgia in addition to this. Not only would you be faced with pain and stiffness in your knee, but the fibromy-algia would cause pain in the neck, back, shoulders, arms, legs, and hips; widespread stiffness accompanied by fatigue; depression; and headache.

It is also fairly common to see fibromyalgia in patients with rheumatoid arthritis. In fact, studies show that more than 20 percent of persons with rheumatoid arthritis also have fibro-myalgia. Rheumatoid arthritis causes chronic pain and swell-ing in the joints of the hands, wrists, elbows, shoulders, knees, ankles, feet, and other joints. Other symptoms include morn-ing stiffness and fatigue. Although some patients definitely have rheumatoid arthritis, they also have all of the typical findings of fibromyalgia. Other forms of arthritis commonly occur along with fibromyalgia, including osteoarthritis, sys-temic lupus erythematosus (SLE or lupus), psoriatic arthritis, or polymyalgia rheumatica. Having one type of arthritis does not prevent you from also developing fibromyalgia!

The disease can also happen in patients who have chronic back pain, injuries to the back or neck, or a ruptured lumbar or cervical disc, as well as internal organ diseases.

Fibromyalgia Increases Depression

As sufferers live with the symptoms of fibromyalgia, they can become more and more focused on their pain and sadness, which is very real. The many appointments with health care providers to try to find relief, combined with the cost of these attempts, add to the patient's frustration.

As time goes on, patients have trouble keeping a job because of their many absences. As income declines, there can be more financial stresses to be dealt with by the sufferer and family. These stresses, along with the constant fatigue, pain, and low-grade depression, can cause severe relationship problems in the family.

The longer the situation lasts, the more likely a patient will see signs of stress, including:

Constant tiredness
Difficulty concentrating
Increasing irritability
Withdrawal from other activities (especially enjoyable
    ones)
Change in appetite
Depression

Each of us shows stress in different ways. If you have been diagnosed with fibromyalgia or think that you may have this disease, it is important to try to understand the ways in which you show stress that accompanies the disease. Then you can begin steps to control the stress (see chapters 5 and 6).

The Cost of Fibromyalgia

In addition to the human cost in suffering to the patient and family, the expenses associated with this disease can be devastating. Health care and medication costs can run to many thousands of dollars, not including the costs of specialized tests, counseling, or hospitalization.

After an extended course of treatment with little control of pain and more loss of activity, patients may be referred to a pain clinic. An inpatient pain clinic with a four-to-six-week treatment can be helpful, but this alone may cost $20,000 or more.

The good news is that large savings in health care costs are possible if the symptoms can be controlled. And the improvement in human costs could affect millions of people.

Take a Proactive Approach to Healing

The fact is, the outlook for people with fibromyalgia is remarkably better than ever before. Ongoing research and scientific trials are providing new information on the disease and how to treat the symptoms successfully. However, the first step in controlling these symptoms is understanding all you can about the disease, including the recommended modes of treatment and seeking a proper diagnosis, which is explained in chapter 2. Most patients feel a noticeable decrease in pain and fatigue and an increase in mobility and energy within a few months of starting treatment. This is exactly what happened to Helen, who has lived with this mysterious disease for two years.

This young attorney told of having throbbing muscle pain when she was in law school. "I was so stressed all the time from trying to compete in my class that I just assumed that the pain and tiredness I felt were caused by this," she told me. "But when I left law school and joined a large practice in town, I continued to have the same symptoms."

Helen lived with undiagnosed fibromyalgia and quietly suffered its life-stealing symptoms—working her school schedule around daily nap periods and avoiding heavy activity or sports for fear of more pain and fatigue. Today she is a different person. She has learned that although the symptoms still wax and wane, she can actively tackle these symptoms with lifestyle changes that make a difference in how she feels each day.

Everyone Is Different

Remember, each person is different. The more specific the diagnosis of arthritis and rheumatic diseases, the more specific the treatment can be. This book cannot replace a proper medical diagnosis. It was written to help you become more informed about fibromyalgia so that you can knowledgeably seek a professional diagnosis from your doctor and begin treatment.

2 MAKING THE DIAGNOSIS

Maria came to see me after living with undiagnosed chronic muscle pain for more than six years. At age thirty-seven, this mother of three told of sleeping all morning after getting her children off to school, taking another late afternoon nap while her children watched TV, then going to bed before 8:00 P.M. When she wasn't sleeping, Maria described symptoms of chronic headache, irritable bowel syndrome, muscle tension, and tender areas that were painful when anyone touched her.

After ruling out other diseases, Maria was diagnosed with fibromyalgia. Even though she realized that there was no cure for this disease, Maria was relieved to know finally what was causing her daily discomfort and fatigue.

Another patient, Susan, had to face a great deal of anger that it had taken so long to make a diagnosis of her chronic sleep problems, depression, and muscle pain. "If I had known then what I know now, I wouldn't have spent more than two thousand dollars trying to find an answer. Half the battle of winning with this disease is knowing that you didn't make it up."

A Difficult Diagnosis

Many patients like Maria and Susan tell of traveling from doctor to doctor with fibromyalgia—without results—because there are no specific tests for the disease. It may be difficult to make an accurate diagnosis if you cannot see a scientific measurement, such as laboratory tests or X rays. This is why in years past, millions of cases were misdiagnosed as depression or chronic fatigue syndrome (CFS).

Normal Laboratory Tests

With today's high-tech medicine, we have become used to special testing, blood tests, or other expensive tests to arrive at a diagnosis. However, most laboratory tests are not very helpful by themselves in making the diagnosis of fibromyalgia. In fact, this is one medical problem in which talking with the patient may be the most important tool in arriving at the correct diagnosis. The reason for this is that the major points for diagnosis of fibromyalgia are discovered from the way that you feel. While a physical examination will show your doctor the painful trigger points, as discussed on page 41, even with trigger points, you must *tell* your doctor of the exact pain you feel in those areas.

Upon evaluation, your doctor will want to have a few basic laboratory tests taken to be sure no other serious medical problems are present. But these tests are limited in number and can be performed at your doctor's office or your local laboratory. They can usually all be done at one visit.

Specific Laboratory Tests Used

Some specific blood tests that your doctor may ask for include a complete blood count (CBC). This test measures hemoglobin levels and provides a count of red blood cells, white blood cells, and platelets. It is used to diagnose many common blood disorders, such as anemia, that can cause fatigue.

The chemistries in your blood will also be checked and will include blood tests that tell how the kidney and liver are functioning, cholesterol and other fats in the blood, calcium levels, and tests of other chemicals such as glucose, that can create problems similar to fibromyalgia, but which are treated differently. Thyroid tests will be done at the same time with blood tests to see if the thyroid is working properly.

Testing for Arthritis

If arthritis is a question, one test that may be included is the *erythrocyte sedimentation rate* (sed rate or ESR). This is an old test that measures the rate at which red blood cells settle out in a tube of unclotted blood; a higher than normal sed rate indicates inflammation. Patients with rheumatoid arthritis and other similar types of arthritis have abnormal sed rates. Patients with osteoarthritis and fibromyalgia, however, usually have normal sed rates. Some infections can also cause an abnormal sed rate; the test is not specific for any one disease.

Your doctor may also ask for another blood test to look for *rheumatoid factor*. Rheumatoid factor is an abnormal protein in the blood present in 70 to 80 percent of patients with rheumatoid arthritis. However, rheumatoid factor can also be present in otherwise normal persons.

Your doctor also may test for *antinuclear antibody* (ANA). Like the rheumatoid factor, ANA is an abnormal protein in the blood and is most commonly found with systemic lupus erythematosus. Lupus is a type of arthritis more commonly found in women, especially younger women. It can cause pain and fatigue, and may also cause internal organ problems, such as kidney disease, heart disease, or problems in the brain.

More than 90 percent of patients with lupus have a positive blood test for antinuclear antibody. However, the test can be positive in persons who do not have lupus or who have other, unrelated diseases. The ANA test is important, but there are usually other clues present as well for your doctor.

X Rays Show No Abnormality

X rays of the painful areas will show no abnormality, because the pain caused by fibromyalgia is in the soft tissues (muscles and tendons), which do not show up well on routine X rays. If you have another problem, such as arthritis, then there may be some abnormalities on the X rays to indicate what type of arthritis is present. Keep in mind that fibromyalgia does not cause X-ray changes.

It is important that you talk openly with your doctor in order to interpret the overall results of the total work-up, including the physical examination, laboratory testing, and X rays. This will allow you to have a good understanding of your problems and will provide the basis for your knowledge of the plan of treatment. At this time, be certain to ask any questions and even ask for printed information to read, if you feel the need.

Trust your doctor to decide which set of tests is best in your case to ensure no other medical problems are present. This can help you avoid extra testing that will add little to your diagnosis and only add expense. If there is one specific diagnosis you fear, such as cancer, be sure you tell your doctor. If you still do not feel comfortable with the diagnosis, talk to your doctor and have more testing. Or get a second opinion until you have peace of mind that the problem has been diagnosed correctly. At that time, proper treatment can begin.

Diagnostic Guidelines

Once other medical problems have been ruled out by laboratory tests and X rays, making the diagnosis of fibromyalgia may still be difficult. There are, however, some other guide-lines and diagnostic criteria physicians use to determine the problem.

1. History of widespread pain for at least three months
   Pain in left side of body
   Pain in right side of body
   Pain above waist
   Pain below waist

In addition, pain must be present in one of the following areas:
   neck (cervical spine)
   front of the chest (anterior chest)
   middle of the back (thoracic spine)
   lower back (lumbar spine)

2. Pain in eleven of eighteen tender or trigger point sites on examination
   The locations of the tender point sites are shown in figure 2.1. These are areas of localized tenderness, much more tender than the surrounding areas. They are often present at tendons, in the soft tissues over bones, and in muscles.

Patients have fibromyalgia if criteria from both classification lists 1 and 2 are present. If a patient has another type of arthritis, she may still be classified as having fibromyalgia if she fulfills criteria from both 1 and 2. For example, it is common for a patient with rheumatoid arthritis or systemic lupus erythematosus also to be diagnosed with fibromyalgia due to generalized pain and tenderness. Once fibromyalgia is diagnosed, treatments are available to help the pain, which are separate from treatments for the other chronic diseases.

Figure 2.1. Trigger areas are tender points over the neck, shoulder blades, lower back, elbows, and knees or other areas. At least eleven of the eighteen trigger points are found to be painful in patients with fibromyalgia.

Diagnosing Fibromyalgia

As your physician makes the diagnosis of fibromyalgia, there are three primary areas that will be considered:

1. Evaluating widespread pain
2. Evaluating trigger points
3. Eliminating other diseases

To be thorough with a diagnosis of fibromyalgia, the following six evaluations are important:

EVALUATE WIDESPREAD PAIN

As explained in chapter 1, patients tell of feeling pain "everywhere," or at least in so many places that it seems to be everywhere. The pain can be sharp, dull, aching, sticking, or pressurelike, or it may be difficult to characterize. The pain often comes from deep within the muscles or joints, as well as from the tendons and ligaments around the joints. Quite often people mistake this pain for a type of true arthritis because of the discomfort and stiffness.

However, the pain from fibromyalgia seems to be from *around* the joints more often than from the joints themselves. Unlike the pain that you may feel after engaging in exercise or a day of housecleaning, which goes away after you walk around, patients tell of pain being present twenty-four hours a day. It makes itself known in the morning on arising and stays all day, even worsening as the day goes on.

Pain is typically felt in the back, neck, arms, and legs, including the shoulders and elbows as well as the hips and buttocks. There may also be pain felt in the hands, wrists, knees, ankles, and feet. Pain in the head and jaws can cause headaches.

Temporomandibular joint syndrome. The most common cause of pain in the jaw and nearby areas of the face and neck has been called temporomandibular joint syndrome (TMJ syndrome). Pain can be felt in the joint itself just in front of the ear, or it might be felt in the side of the face, head, or neck. There is usually tenderness to the touch in the jaw muscles around the joint. You may also feel a sensation of cracking in the jaw when the mouth is opened. This jaw pain can happen alone from muscle tenderness, or it can be part of fibromyalgia.

With TMJ, the pain may be constant, it may worsen with

chewing or when you open your jaw. Headaches are common along with the jaw pain, since the jaw pain may be felt all over the side of the head and neck. There may be tender points and points that trigger off pain in other areas when they are examined by your doctor.

Widespread pain felt all over. Pain is also commonly felt in the abdomen, along with cramps, diarrhea, and constipation. Pain in the bladder area, along with frequent urination, is common. Menstrual periods may be much more painful than usual. Pain may be felt in the chest and may be difficult to tell from pain due to heart disease.

The American College of Rheumatology found that almost all fibromyalgia patients have widespread pain above the waist, below the waist, on the right and left sides of their bodies, and in the neck or back areas. Indeed, people with fibromyalgia may have more pain receptors than others or might be overly sensitive to everything. One patient said just taking a warm bubble bath was a painful experience. The symptom of widespread pain is important in making an accurate diagnosis and in telling the difference between fibromyalgia and other problems.

Understanding acute and chronic pain. Acute pain is important, because it brings to your attention a problem that might cause damage to the body. Acute pain could be a toothache from a cavity, a broken bone, a headache from a sinus infection, or a backache from a strain. Muscle pain, joint pain, and pain in the stomach could all be acute signals of a potential problem. Some injuries can cause acute pain, such as the pain associated with bursitis and tendinitis. Each of these types of acute pain runs its course and disappears as the problem is relieved.

Surveys have shown that more than 70 percent of Americans have acute pain from headache at some time each year, and more than 50 percent have backaches. These pains usually last a few days to weeks. When the problem is relieved, or the injury heals, the pain leaves. For example, acute back pain, the most common cause of loss of work except for the common cold, can come on suddenly and can be severe, but in more than 80 percent of cases it goes away in about two weeks.

Researchers consider acute pain that lasts one to six months longer than expected to be *chronic,* depending on the problem that causes the pain. For example, a back injury causes acute pain; if the pain is no better after three months, it is called chronic back pain. Pain that returns over and over for months or years can be considered chronic. Back pain that is severe and returns many times over one or more years is called chronic back pain. Pain from fibromyalgia is chronic; it lasts for at least three months.

Finding underlying problems.   Internal organ problems can cause chronic pain that may mimic the overall aching or throbbing muscle pain of fibromyalgia. If the pain is caused by kidney disease, stomach disease, or other internal organ abnormality, correcting the basic problem will remove the pain. Thus, it is necessary to find and treat any underlying causes of pain before starting treatment for what may seem to be pain from fibromyalgia.

For example, Colleen, a forty-seven-year-old woman, had chronic back pain for more than six months. She had been evaluated for ruptured lumbar disc, but the tests were negative. At that point, she read about fibromyalgia and immediately assumed that this was the proper diagnosis for her pain. However, further testing showed that she actually had a problem with gallbladder disease. After surgery on the gallbladder, her chronic back pain went away completely.

Another middle-aged woman came to our clinic with pain in the lower back and hip area that had lasted for months and had gradually become worse. When it began keeping her awake for several nights in a row, she became worried and sought further help. She was found to have cancer that had spread to the bones of the spine. After starting immediate treatment, she was free of pain.

EVALUATE TRIGGER POINTS

In 1990, the American College of Rheumatology established specific diagnostic criteria that require the presence of specific tender or trigger points that are painful to touch when pushed or palpated. In fact, these trigger points are key diagnostic features of the disease (see figure 2.1).

Trigger points, as discussed in chapter 1, are small, localized areas in muscles and tendons that are very tender to pressure in persons with fibromyalgia. These trigger areas are much more sensitive than other nearby areas. In fact, pressure on one of the trigger points with a finger causes pain that makes the person flinch or pull back. The actual size of a trigger point is usually very small, about the size of a penny. Trigger points are scattered over the neck, back, chest, elbows, hips, buttocks, and knees (see figure 2.1), and eleven or more of these are found in most patients with fibromyalgia.

In some conditions other than fibromyalgia, trigger-point pain may be felt in areas away from the actual tender trigger point. For example, pain may seem to travel down one or both legs when trigger areas are pushed in the lower back. This can mimic the pain of pressure on a nerve in the lower back from a ruptured disc, called *sciatica.*

When a physician tests trigger points for pain, he or she will also check *control points* or other nontender points on the body to make sure the person does not react to these as well, which would change the diagnosis. Some physicians use a special instrument, called a *doximeter* or *dolorimeter*, to apply just the right amount of pressure on trigger points.

ASK ABOUT FATIGUE

Fatigue has been estimated by researchers to be present at any one time in up to 25 percent of all of us. It can be mild and easily cured by getting extra rest and sleep. But fatigue, tiredness, and exhaustion can be prolonged (lasting more than one month) or chronic (lasting more than six months).

ASSESS YOUR LEVEL OF FATIGUE

Fatigue prevents you from doing normal activities and chores

You have difficulty making plans due to unpredictable fatigue

Fatigue is still there after rest or at least eight hours of sleep

Fatigue interferes with work outside the home

Fatigue hinders relationship with family members and friends

You have difficulty getting through the day because of fatigue

Fatigue prevents exercise or other activity

This loss of energy is the major complaint of most patients with fibromyalgia and may cause more limitation than the pain. Many patients tell us that if it were not for the fatigue, they could put up with the pain of fibromyalgia.

The fatigue associated with fibromyalgia severely limits daily activities. The tiredness may be especially bothersome in the morning and then improve after a few hours, only to return later in the day. There may be a window of time in each day when activities are tolerated after the morning fatigue wears off but before the afternoon fatigue hits again.

Patients tell of fatigue being most noticeable during activity, which causes immobility as the fatigue becomes more limiting. Fatigue can be even more severe following exercise—it may last days and be so worrisome that a person becomes sedentary.

Fatigue may be worse when a person is physically deconditioned—out of shape. For example, if physical activity has been avoided for a long enough period of time, muscle weakness or tiredness may by itself contribute to fatigue. Researchers have shown that most fibromyalgia patients have below average fitness levels compared to other persons, and when these people do exercise, they complain of sore muscles without much effort. Many patients with fibromyalgia feel too tired even to work, creating large disability and compensation costs for their employers.

Another condition that can be hard to distinguish from fibromyalgia and causes severe fatigue is *chronic fatigue syndrome* (CFS). In this condition, fatigue lasts more than six months, interfering with daily activities both at home and at work, with no medical problem to explain it.

COMMON SYMPTOMS OF CHRONIC FATIGUE SYNDROME
Relentless fatigue
Memory and concentration problems
Sore throat
Swollen lymph nodes
Muscle and joint pains
Headaches
Poor sleep that is not restful
Exhaustion after exercise

A recent study from the American College of Rheumatology suggests that fibromyalgia and chronic fatigue syndrome may even overlap in the same person. With both conditions, the fatigue and other symptoms seem to increase after periods of high stress or physical exertion. Other studies have indicated that many people who were initially diagnosed as having chronic fatigue syndrome probably have fibromyalgia. After some of these patients started the specific treatment for fibromyalgia, their symptoms lessened dramatically and their energy levels increased.

It may be hard to distinguish between fibromyalgia and chronic fatigue syndrome, as some patients with fibromyalgia tell of symptoms, listed above, that are similar to those of

CFS. However, chronic fatigue syndrome patients usually have fever and swollen lymph nodes, and the onset of the problem is more sudden. Also, CFS patients don't usually have prominent trigger points of pain.

Your doctor can help you decide what your fatigue indicates, but other medical problems that cause fatigue need to be evaluated and eliminated.

INQUIRE ABOUT SLEEP DISTURBANCES

Almost all patients with fibromyalgia complain of sleep disturbances. They tell of waking up frequently during the night and feeling tired and unrefreshed during the day; many require more frequent rest periods during the day. Some researchers find that it may be the constant pain that interrupts sleep.

There is some evidence that sleep disturbances may be caused by an abnormality of deep sleep. Patients tell of feeling awake or in a shallow state of sleep throughout the night, instead of experiencing restful, deep-level sleep. FMS patients also show abnormal brain waveforms in deep sleep. Unfortunately, it is during the delta, or deep-level, sleep that the body does its repair work and replenishment. The hormone *somatostatin,* for example, which is produced in deep sleep and is vital for maintaining good muscle and other soft tissue health, has been found at low levels in fibromyalgia patients. If deep sleep is reduced over a long period of time, the body may have less ability to repair and replenish energy.

ASSESS SLEEP PROBLEMS
Many arousals during a night's sleep
Awakening in the middle of the night
Difficulty in getting to sleep
Reduction in total sleep time
Long awakenings (ten minutes or more) during sleep
Restless legs syndrome during sleep

EVALUATE STRESS LEVEL

Evaluating the patient's lifestyle and work habits to see if she is experiencing undue stress or uneasiness each day is an important factor in making a diagnosis. However, which came first: stress or fibromyalgia?

Doctors know that the stress of living with unending, throbbing, or stabbing pain and relentless fatigue can put the patient into overload, resulting in overwhelming feelings of nervousness and anxiety. But they are uncertain as to which came first—a stressful life that brings about the fibromyalgia syndrome or whether having this disease leads to the stress. One study tested fibromyalgia patients on the Hospital Anxiety and Depression Index and a startling 92 percent of patients had a high score. Some consider fibromyalgia to be a psychosomatic illness in which psychological problems, such as depression, disappointment, and anxiety express themselves as physical symptoms, such as backache and sore muscles.

STRESSORS WITH FIBROMYALGIA
Physical stressors (the pain)
Social stressors (loss of friends and activities)
Work stressors (loss of job or difficulty working)
Family stressors (feeling of dependency on others)

No matter which came first, stress can add to problems of anger, distractibility, and irritability and can even lead to further physical changes, such as hypertension or cardiac problems.

ASSESS LEVEL OF STRESS
Various physical symptoms stemming from stress
Feeling overwhelmed day after day
Anxiety upon awakening
Impatient for no apparent reason
Unable to sleep soundly

Difficulty in concentrating on projects at home or work
Loss of interest or enjoyment in life
Easy to anger or frequent irritability
Changes in appetite (eating more or less food)

TEST FOR DEPRESSION

"I don't know if I'm depressed because I ache all over or because I am clinically depressed," Britt said. "I'm not used to being restricted in what I can do and feel caged in by this disease, as if it has a hold on me and won't let me feel free to move like I used to."

Britt told of depression lingering day after day, even when she had everything going for her. She had two healthy children and a husband who was supportive. "Every day I think that maybe this is the day that the sadness will lift. But after tossing and turning each night, I only awaken to more pain and sadness. Will it ever end?"

Again, which came first, fibromyalgia or depression? That question continues to puzzle many researchers, who have found that the two illnesses have similar characteristics. Many people with fibromyalgia are depressed. Conversely, depressed people often complain of inexplainable aches and pains along with fatigue and an inability to stay asleep at night. At some point researchers find depression present in the majority of fibromyalgia patients. In fact, *more than 25 percent* of patients do have depression when fibromyalgia is diagnosed.

When evaluating a patient, the doctor will talk about feelings of depression, as listed below.

COMMON SIGNALS OF DEPRESSION

Disturbances in sleep patterns
Loss of interest in usual activities
Weight loss or gain (more than 5 percent of body weight)
Fatigue
Impaired thinking
Thoughts of dying or suicide

Depressed thoughts or irritability
Mood swings
Staying at home all the time
Avoidance of special friends
Difficulty concentrating
Feelings of worthlessness or excessive or inappropriate
  guilt
Agitation or, in contrast, a general slowing of intentional
  bodily activity

Living with the constant pain and fatigue of fibromyalgia can bring about feelings of depression with hopelessness, uncontrollable tearfulness, loss of self-worth, and even suicidal thoughts. Some normal individuals may have one or more symptoms of depression at one time or another. Depression becomes a problem when symptoms begin to occur on a daily basis for a period of at least two weeks and are accompanied by other feelings, such as the fatigue, pain, and muscle aches.

Depression is a very complicated affliction and is not as easy to deal with as other worries and stressors mentioned in this chapter. Often, depression can stem from a biochemical imbalance or can be a symptom of an underlying ailment. Quite often professional help is needed to maintain, control, and cure depression. There are many excellent prescription drugs and many medical protocols that can assist greatly in controlling depression.

Fibromyalgia Can Be Discouraging

These are the most common feelings and signs of fibromyalgia your doctor may consider as he or she makes an accurate diagnosis. I know that these symptoms can be discouraging. The constant muscle pain and fatigue can make daily activities, such as standing, walking, sitting, and even coughing, unbearable. See figure 2.2.

Pain and fatigue lead to inactivity. Because of the disrupted sleep patterns and failure to receive much needed restful sleep, the patient is fatigued even on arising. Daily fatigue can lead to personality changes. A once calm individual will now have a low frustration level, making it difficult to get along at home or work.

With the constant pain and feeling of exhaustion, it is no wonder the patient feels depressed. This in turn can lead to further feelings of discouragement and may create additional social problems and withdrawal from normal activities. Depression may worsen if certain medications, such as tranquilizers to aid with sleep, are used—especially if taken too frequently.

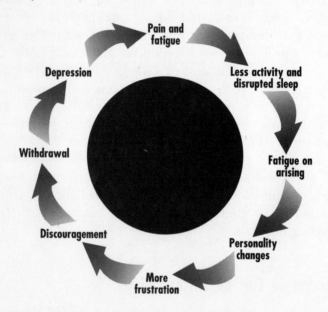

Figure 2.2. Cycle of depression with fibromyalgia.

The 7-Step Treatment Program Does Work

The earlier the 7-Step Treatment Program is started, the better the chances are of improvement in a patient's symptoms. The program involves:

1. Experimenting with medications and treatments until a protocol that works is established.
2. Doing specific exercises to reduce muscle pain and increase strength and energy.
3. Learning ways to de-stress and alleviate anxiety at home and in the workplace.
4. Trying a complementary approach to reducing symptoms, including Chinese medicine therapies, homeopathy, chiropractic, acupuncture, massage and therapeutic touch, biofeedback, and herbal therapy, among others.
5. Learning ways to enhance restful sleep and understanding the serotonin/fibromyalgia connection.
6. Starting a nutritional plan for healing using phytochemicals and antioxidants.
7. Understanding the importance of support for symptom relief.

The next seven chapters explain each of these important treatment modalities and, if followed, will enable you to overcome the disabling effects of fibromyalgia.

3

STEP 1: START WITH MEDICAL TREATMENT

Jacqueline's experience was quite typical of most patients'. She started out with excruciating pain upon arising one morning. She assumed this was a lingering symptom from the flu. Her doctor prescribed an over-the-counter pain medication and told her to drink plenty of fluids and get rest. This thirty-six-year-old interior decorator told of staying in bed for two weeks, putting clients on hold, and farming her children out to friends while trying to get well.

"When I was no better two weeks later," she told me, "I knew I was up against something far worse than the winter flu." Jacqueline went from doctor to doctor, all of whom drew blood for lab work and took many X rays, but to no avail.

"When the last doctor sat me down and went over my chart, he looked at me and said, 'I cannot find anything wrong. You are a well person.' That did it! I knew I was not well, but I was determined to get well."

Jacqueline was diagnosed with fibromyalgia after going over her list of symptoms, including overall deep muscle pain, inability to sleep at night, depression, dizziness, irritable bowel syndrome, urinary frequency, painful menstrual cramps, and headaches. She was put on the 7-Step Treatment Program outlined in this book. While she is not cured—as there is no cure for this disease—she does have more good days than bad days and is able to function and do the things she wants to without debilitating symptoms.

If you have fibromyalgia and live with constant pain and fatigue, like millions of other sufferers, you have probably tried many ways to obtain relief. But to control the pain and other symptoms, you need a multidisciplinary approach. Each step described in the 7-Step Treatment Program is used in conjunction with the others and should be adapted to your lifestyle on a daily basis. Again, the steps will not cure the disease, but they will curb the symptoms.

Start with Moist Heat

Perhaps you have already tried a heating pad at times and found some relief for your aching muscles. I want you to carry this therapy further and use moist heat, twice daily, for ten to twenty minutes on areas of your body that have pain. Twice daily, every day without fail helps relax tense muscles, which makes exercising easier and relieves pain and more.

Because most patients complain of pain all over the body, the most effective and easy-to-use forms of moist heat are a warm shower, hot tub bath, whirlpool, or heated swimming pool. For example, it is easy to put a chair or stool (with rubber tips on the legs for safety) in the shower, then let the warm water permeate the back. Or, if you have access to a whirlpool bath or spa, use it twice daily. Some patients alternate the whirlpool and shower until they find one that is most effective. A warm bath may work for your overall pain, especially the legs and back, but with chronic pain, it may be difficult to sit and then get up from the tub.

If the pain is so intense that you cannot use the shower, whirlpool, or bathtub, then use warm, moist towels or a moist heating pad. Just put the moist towels on the back for a few minutes and change them for warm ones when they cool off.

Another choice is hot packs, which can be purchased at a medical supply store. These are heated in hot water, wrapped in a towel, and placed on the back. Some packs are available that can be warmed in a microwave oven. These may be easier to use, but don't allow them to get too hot to touch.

INDIVIDUAL CHOICE OF TREATMENT

You may ignore every treatment suggestion in this book, but DO NOT IGNORE using moist heat, twice daily. The relief from pain that you will feel will make it worth the small about of time you sacrifice each day.

Choose the form of moist heat that is most convenient and works best for you. Then plan to use it regularly every day. You may quickly find a reduction in pain that will last for a few minutes or hours. Mary Catherine told me emphatically that moist heat did nothing to relieve her pain, but upon questioning, she told me she only used it during her daily shower for ten minutes. Once she began a twice daily program, she experienced pain relief and was virtually sold on this part of the treatment program.

HELPFUL FORMS OF MOIST HEAT FOR FIBROMYALGIA PAIN
Heated swimming pool
Warm whirlpool or hot tub
Warm shower
Warm tub bath
Hot packs
Warm, moist towel or cloth
Moist heating pad

Add Medications

Certain medications are an effective part of the treatment program for fibromyalgia, along with the twice daily use of moist heat. Medications can provide much needed relief of the pain and deep, throbbing muscle aches. In our clinic, we encourage patients to use the lowest dosage possible of any medication and to find the medication that has the fewest side effects. Try to be patient. If pain relief is not experienced with the first medications you try, you and your physician may have to try other combinations.

If you notice unusual symptoms or side effects, stop taking the medication and talk to your doctor.

TRY ANTIDEPRESSANT MEDICATIONS IN FIBROMYALGIA

The most helpful medicines are from a group of prescription drugs also used to treat depression, specifically tricyclic and tetracyclic antidepressant drugs. These are examples of medicines that can be used for more than one purpose. The rationale for their use is twofold—most increase the time spent in stage 4 sleep, and they increase the amount of serotonin in the central nervous system, which has a calming effect (see pages 74 and 75). You may want to discuss with your doctor the fact that these are used for depression.

Amitriptyline (Elavil) is one of the most commonly used of these medications. It is one of the oldest antidepressants and has been shown to work well in about one-third of patients. Another bonus is that amitriptyline is very inexpensive. Keep in mind that in fibromyalgia, amitriptyline is used in much lower doses than commonly used for depression. Also, a word of caution: In older people, this medication is usually avoided because of the possible side effects discussed below.

If amitriptyline does not work or has side effects, there are other similar medications to try. Some of the most common are listed on pages 54 and 55. Be patient during this process of elimination, as it may take two or three weeks before any improvement is shown. You may need to try a number of these medications before you find one that works best for you. However, when you find the right one, you'll know it. There will be a definite reduction of pain, stiffness, and fatigue, and your sleep quality will improve.

Your goal should be to choose the medication that gives the greatest relief with the least side effects. About 30 to 60 percent of FMS patients find that one of these medications gives enough improvement that they want to continue taking the drug.

If one of these medications does not give relief of pain and fatigue, there are some newer medications used for treatment of depression that are used in fibromyalgia. These newer medications treat depression by increasing the effect of serotonin, which is thought to be low in fibromyalgia. In most cases, newer medications have fewer side effects than the older antidepressant drugs routinely used. Nonetheless, it may take a few weeks to feel an effect on pain and fatigue. And it may still be necessary to try several of the group to see which gives the best effect without side effects.

In some cases your doctor may combine more than one of these medications to try to maximize the positive effect without side effects caused by high doses. Make it your goal to find the right combination that gives improvement in pain and improvement in activity without side effects.

Side effects are usually few if lower doses of the medicines are used. The most common side effects are drowsiness (which may help improve the quality of sleep when taken at night), dryness in the mouth, constipation (which is usually not serious), or occasional difficulty in urination. Less common side effects are dizziness, blurred vision, rapid heart rate, or confusion. If you also take other medication, check with your doctor to make sure there are no unwanted problems from the combination of drugs.

SOME OF THE MOST COMMONLY USED ANTIDEPRESSANTS IN FIBROMYALGIA
Ascendin
Desyrel
Effexor
Elavil
Norpramin

Pamelor
Paxil
Prozac
Remeron
Serzone
Sinequan
Surmontil
Tofranil
Wellbutrin
Zoloft

NONSTEROIDAL ANTI-INFLAMMATORY DRUGS

Often, nonsteroidal anti-inflammatory drugs (NSAIDs) are given to patients with fibromyalgia. Since there is little inflammation with the disease, these drugs usually are not very effective. But these medications can also have some pain-relieving *(analgesic)* effect that may give relief at times. If you don't find relief from pain after about two weeks, try a different nonsteroidal anti-inflammatory drug or acetaminophen (such as Tylenol), which is not a NSAID and is well tolerated by asthmatics and people with gastrointestinal problems.

SOME COMMON NONSTEROIDAL ANTI-INFLAMMATORY DRUGS

TRADE NAME	GENERIC NAME
Advil	ibuprofen
Aleve	naproxen
Anaprox	naproxen
Ansaid	flurbiprofen
Arthrotec	diclofenac plus misoprostol
Aspirin products	acetylsalicyclic acid
Clinoril	sulindac
Daypro	oxaprozin
Disalcid	salsalate
Dolobid	diflunisal

TRADE NAME	GENERIC NAME
Feldene	piroxicam
Indocin	indomethacin
Lodine	etodolac
Magan	magnesium salicylate
Meclomen	meclofenamate
Monogesic	salsalate
Motrin	ibuprofen
Nalfon	fenoprofen
Naprelan	naproxen sodium
Naprosyn	naproxen
Orudis	ketoprofen
Oruvail	ketoprofen
Relafen	nabumetone
Salflex	salsalate
Tolectin	tolmetin
Trilisate	choline magnesium trisalicylate
Voltaren	diclofenac sodium
Zorprin	zero-order release aspirin (12-hour)

If these drugs give relief, they can be used for a long period of time, but you must always watch for side effects, especially for any upset stomach, since development of peptic ulcers are a possibility. Other serious side effects include dark, sticky bowel movements and blood in the stool. About 1 percent of those who take these NSAIDs for six months or longer have blood in their stool.

THE NEW SUPER ASPIRINS
If you rely on traditional nonsteroidal anti-inflammatory drugs (NSAIDs)—Advil, aspirin, Motrin, naprosyn—to help ease the deep muscle pain of fibromyalgia, you know how these can often cause stomach distress. NSAIDs work by slowing

the action of prostaglandins. These are the chemicals that cause inflammation in arthritis. But prostaglandins also have a positive benefit of protecting the stomach from irritation. Up to now, the available NSAIDs slowed both the bad and good prostaglandins.

The new COX-2 inhibitors or "super aspirins" work in a different way than the older NSAIDs. They stop the "bad" prostaglandins that cause pain and inflammation, while allowing the "good" prostaglandins to do their job protecting your stomach from peptic ulcers. Ask your doctor if one of these new medications would help you.

NEW SUPER ASPIRINS
Celebrex

Mobic

Vioxx

You will need to have a blood test taken every few months to check for side effects. If you have any questions, talk to your doctor before you continue to take any NSAIDs.

COMMONLY USED H2 BLOCKERS
(OVER-THE-COUNTER MEDICATIONS THAT BLOCK ACID PRODUCTION)

TRADE NAME	GENERIC NAME
Axid	nizatidine
Pepcid AC	famotidine
Tagamet	cimetidine
Zantac	ranitidine

PRESCRIPTION MEDICATIONS THAT BLOCK ACID PRODUCTION

TRADE NAME	GENERIC NAME
Prevacid	lausoprazole
Prilosec	omeprazole

SOME OF THE MOST COMMON SIDE EFFECTS OF NSAIDS

Abdominal pain
Abnormal liver tests (blood tests)
Allergic or unusual reactions
Anemia (lower hemoglobin)
Asthma in those allergic
Blurred vision (occasional)
Confusion
Constipation
Decreased platelet count (can affect bleeding)
Depression
Diarrhea
Difficulty sleeping
Diminished effect of diuretics
Dizziness
Fatigue
Gastritis
Headaches
Heartburn
Hypertension (increased blood pressure)
Impaired thinking (uncommon, but occurs at times in
    older people)
Indigestion
Intestinal bleeding
Itching
Lowered white cells in blood count
Meningitis-like illness (rare)
Mouth ulcers
Palpitations
Peptic ulcers
Rash
Renal (kidney) failure
Sleepiness
Sodium retention with edema (swelling)
Sun sensitivity
Tinnitus (ringing in the ears)

CORTISONE-TYPE DRUGS

Cortisone-type drugs are almost never given regularly by mouth to fibromyalgia patients, as the side effects of long-term use are not worth the benefits. On the other hand, local injections of a cortisone derivative into a painful trigger point can be used. This type of injection is usually combined with a local anesthetic and can give good relief from pain at the particular trigger point that may last from weeks to months (see page 68).

MUSCLE RELAXANTS

Many patients find temporary relief for back and neck pain with such muscle relaxants as cyclobenzaprine (Flexeril), chlorzoxazone (Parafon Forte), methocarbamol (Robaxin), or carisoprodol (Soma). The benefit of muscle relaxants is that they can be used as needed, since they usually give rapid relief that lasts for a few hours. If they don't, then they should be eliminated.

In some clinical tests of FMS patients, Flexeril has been shown to be effective in relieving muscle pain. Although it may work in only 30 to 40 percent of patients, those who find that it helps report getting excellent relief. For those with FMS, Flexeril is often taken at bedtime.

Side effects of muscle relaxants are usually not serious. The most common side effect is drowsiness.

NONNARCOTIC PAIN MEDICATIONS

Nonnarcotic prescription pain medicines may give relief for hours and can be used when needed. The advantage of this type of medication is that it may not cause the drowsiness or loss of alertness that narcotics can create and is not habit-forming. It is important to be sure that your activity level is improving when you take any type of pain medicines in fibromyalgia. There is no real advantage in simply killing the pain and remaining inactive.

Most who take one of these medications do not have side effects, yet if you try one of them, make sure the medication does not cause nausea. Nonnarcotic pain medications are intended for short-term use (about ten days or less) unless you discuss it with your doctor, so you can monitor for side effects.

OVER-THE-COUNTER NONNARCOTIC PAIN MEDICATIONS

TRADE NAME	GENERIC NAME
Advil	ibuprofen
Aleve	naproxen
Many brands of aspirin	acetylsalicyclic acid
Tylenol	acetaminophen

Follow directions on the label, and stop the medication if you have abdominal pain or upset stomach. If you have a peptic ulcer, ask your doctor before taking these medications.

NONNARCOTIC PAIN MEDICATIONS

TRADE NAME	GENERIC NAME
Toradol	ketorolac
Ultram	tramadol

NARCOTIC PAIN MEDICATIONS

Narcotic prescription pain medicines are not recommended for regular use in the treatment of fibromyalgia pain, since narcotics can be habit-forming, and it is likely that there will be a need to find a better long-term solution for pain control. Narcotics can aggravate depression, which can be a part of the fibromyalgia patient's problems. However, in occasional cases of fibromyalgia, when pain is not relieved by all other methods, narcotics may be used for pain relief and to allow improvement in activity. Especially with narcotic use for pain, it is important that activity increase along with pain control to justify their use.

Narcotic pain medications commonly cause constipation if taken regularly.

MEDICATIONS FOR ANXIETY

Some medicines may help the anxiety brought on by the constant pain and fatigue or by the stress of living with fibromyalgia. Anxiety may accompany depression when it is found along with fibromyalgia, and anxiety may cause worsening of other feelings of fibromyalgia.

Xanax (alprazolam) is used for anxiety and associated depression. In one study, half of the fibromyalgia patients showed improvement with alprazolam and ibuprofen. Although it may take eight to sixteen weeks to feel the full effect of alprazolam, this combination can be tried, especially if anxiety is a major problem with fibromyalgia. Most persons do not have side effects, but watch for sleepiness or decreased alertness.

MEDICINES FOR RESTFUL SLEEP

Prescription sleeping pills can also aggravate depression and often don't give excellent results in most patients. Your doctor can help you decide if they would be helpful in your own situation.

To induce deep sleep states small doses of Elavil, Sinequan, or Flexeril may be beneficial. Some patients benefit from the over-the-counter supplement melatonin. In the body, this hormone is produced only at night by the pineal gland in the brain. With sunlight, the body's primary timekeeper, this natural hormone helps to set the brain's biological clock. This clock determines all of the body's circadian rhythms, from hormone releases and body temperature to the sleep-wake cycle and digestive functions.

As a natural supplement, melatonin is available over the counter in drugstores or health food stores. It has been cited in the media as a breakthrough for everything from anti-aging and cancer prevention to treatment of sleep disorders. Even though this hormone is *not* regulated by the Food and Drug Administration, it has been recommended by many researchers as a way to counter the effects of jet lag. The National Institutes of Health is sponsoring $50 million of research on melatonin at this time, yet many of these claims will take years to sort out with scientific studies.

In some sleep research studies, scientists report that melatonin taken an hour before bedtime has been shown to induce sleep more quickly and continue longer than with a placebo. Though melatonin appears to be nontoxic, taking too much or at the wrong time could make you sleepy when you need to be awake! For those with fibromyalgia and the relentless fatigue, being sleepy during the daytime is not a desirable side effect.

At this writing, there is very little evidence as to the longterm effects of melatonin or even the doses recommended. If you want to try melatonin, first talk with your doctor. Then, with your doctor's consent, try a low dose (1 mg) until you get an idea of how you might react. Some patients have reported negative side effects such as grogginess upon awakening, daytime drowsiness, depression, and vivid nightmares.

If you do take melatonin, keep in mind that researchers are still concerned about the unknown side effects associated with natural supplements, as well as the possibility of undiscovered health risks. Actually, some newer studies have found that sweat and heat work much better than any sleep aid. Exercise raises the body temperature when performed in the afternoon, and this extra heat allows the body to go into deeper sleep at nighttime. You can get the same effect with "passive heating," or taking a warm bath several hours before you go to sleep at night.

Help or Hype? New and Experimental Methods of Treating Fibromyalgia

With all the medical research, there are many breakthrough medications and treatments for fibromyalgia—some that are accepted by the medical community and some that draw questions.

As you take new medications or proposed "cures," keep in mind that the power of belief in healing is massive. It was once estimated that about one-third of all healing occurred simply because the patient believed the treatment would work. This is called the *placebo effect*. Some researchers theorize that as much as *two-thirds* of all healing occurs because of the patient's positive beliefs. Placebos have been proven effective in relieving the very real symptoms of colds, headaches, seasickness, angina, anxiety, and postoperative pain.

The following new and experimental treatments may be helpful in your situation. Before you try one, talk with your doctor to see if the treatment is effective. Weigh the effectiveness of the treatment with any side effects. You may want to keep a daily journal of symptoms once you begin the treatment to see if it, in fact, really works.

GUAIFENESIN

For the past several years, guaifenesin, a new "cure" for fibromyalgia, has been touted by some physicians. Although there are no published clinical trials or studies in medical journals showing results of a cure, many patients with FMS claim to have found relief taking this medication. Nonetheless, before you run to the corner drugstore and try to find guaifenesin, it's important to know what it is and what it is intended to do in FMS.

Guaifenesin is not a recent medical discovery. Rather, it is an inexpensive expectorant found in many cough remedies. (Robitussin is an over-the-counter cough medication; Humibid is a prescription product.) Guaifenesin has no significant side effects, and for people with bronchial or lung problems it helps to thin mucus, making it easier to expel.

Proponents postulate that in people with FMS, there is an excess accumulation of phosphates. Guaifenesin helps the kidneys excrete and lower the phosphate levels in the blood.

According to those who have tried this medication at the lowest recommended dosage (300 mg, twice a day), symptoms of fibromyalgia intensify during the first few months of treatment, which is said to be a sign of "disease reversal," and then symptoms may subside.

The effects of guaifenesin is said to be blocked by sources of salicylates, including aspirin. If you choose to try this treatment, first talk with your doctor. You may want to follow a strict dietary plan that excludes salicylates from your meals and medications (aspirin), as well as avoid cosmetics and personal hygiene products containing this substance.

Many leading researchers believe that because millions of FMS patients have been told the problems are "mental" in nature, having the hope of a "cure" can give something positive to cling to. Feeling in control of one's health is crucial for wellness, and guaifenesin has given some this type of self-efficacy.

The bottom line is guaifenesin will *not* hurt you and it may help. However, so far, the scientific proof that this medication will cure fibromyalgia is simply not there. Continue to follow your doctor's instructions, report to your regular visits, and ask questions about any highly promoted "cure" for FMS before you opt to use it. On the other hand, if you do find relief with guaifenesin or other nontraditional treatment with no unwanted side effects, more power to you!

NADH

NADH is a naturally occurring enzyme found in all living cells. This enzyme plays a central role in the body's energy-producing capacity. In the past few years, researchers at Georgetown University have treated patients with chronic fatigue syndrome with NADH with promising results. In these clinical trials, patients reported relief from fatigue, along with increased strength and endurance, and a boost in mental and physical energy.

While the jury is still out on the optimal effectiveness of

NADH in symptoms of fatigue and muscle aches, the data on this experimental drug look promising.

DETROL

As discussed, treating symptoms is the best way to control FMS. Overactive bladder, including symptoms of urinary frequency, urgency, or urge incontinence, is a major concern of many. (Urgency is the sudden, overwhelming urge to urinate; frequency means urinating more than eight times in twenty-four hours; and urge incontinence is the sudden and total involuntary loss of urine.)

Recently, the FDA approved Detrol (tolterodine tartrate) tablets for the treatment of overactive bladder. This breakthrough prescription medication is the first new drug approved for a bladder control problem in the United States in more than twenty years.

Many FMS patients tell of having to change their lifestyle to cope with an overactive bladder to the extent of even reducing fluids or staying inside all day and night. In some cases, having an overactive bladder can result in emotional distress and contribute to depression.

Taking 2 milligrams of Detrol, twice a day, patients experienced a significant reduction in frequency of urination. The side effects are minimal but may include dry mouth, headache, constipation, indigestion, and dry eyes.

Ask your doctor if Detrol may help you return to a normal, active life.

MALIC ACID AND SUPER MALIC

In recent years, evidence has been gathered that suggests FMS is the result of local hypoxia to the muscles, meaning patients have low muscle-tissue oxygen pressure in affected muscles. Malic acid, derived from such foods as apples, apricots (both fresh and dried), cherries, plums, and dried dates and figs, may play a key role in energy production, specifically during hypoxic conditions. In some test studies, volunteers with FMS took 1,200 to 2,400 milligrams of malic acid. Within forty-eight hours of supplementation, they had improvement in pain relief. Likewise, upon discontinuation of malic acid for forty-eight hours, the improvement was lost.

Super Malic, a tablet containing malic acid (200 mg) and magnesium (50 mg), is being studied for treatment of fibromyalgia. In scientific studies, volunteers with FMS took a fixed dose of Super Malic. Although no symptom change was seen in short-term trials, when the dose was increased (up to six tablets of Super Malic, twice a day) and continued for a longer duration of treatment in the open label trial, some reductions in the severity of pain and tenderness were found.

Researchers believe that Super Malic is safe and may be helpful in treating FMS. If you try Super Malic with your doctor's consent, consider staying on this therapy for at least two months to receive full benefit.

MAGNET THERAPY

Many with FMS are turning to magnet therapy in an attempt to find treatment for pain without drugs. This form of drugless therapy is used by many athletes and touted for relieving pain within minutes in some cases.

Magnet therapy goes back for centuries. Some believers feel that the magnet stimulates or interacts with the body's electrical system to increase circulation, reduce inflammation, and decrease pain. Others, who faithfully strap magnets onto sore muscles, claim that the magnetic field interferes with the body's pain perception and the magnets stimulate endorphins in the body (natural painkillers).

Quite honestly, no one really knows how magnets work. A surprising study from Baylor College of Medicine recently revealed that magnets may reduce muscular pain in post-polio patients. Volunteers in the Baylor study said they got pain relief from very low energy magnets (300 to 500 gauss or a little larger than a refrigerator magnet)—once a day for only forty-five minutes.

It would take subsequent studies to make any guarantees, yet even some researchers are strapping magnets to arthritic knees in hopes this experimental treatment works. At this time, the National Institutes of Health has created an office of alternative medicine, which is paying for the magnet studies on fibromyalgia patients at the University of Virginia.

The downside of magnet therapy is the unknown. The FDA warns doctors about the unknown side effects of magnet therapy. Just as they do not know if magnets can end pain, they don't know if they are harmful either. Some have reported such side effects as headaches, insomnia, and backache after extensive magnet therapy.

It's important to realize that although there is hope for magnet therapy in stopping chronic pain, it is still highly experimental and if used incorrectly can induce brain seizures in healthy people.

HUMAN GROWTH HORMONE

Some researchers suspect that human growth hormone, a hormone secreted by the pituitary gland in the brain, may be related to fibromyalgia. Studies show lower levels of human growth hormone in patients with FMS, even compared to those who suffered from pain but not fibromyalgia.

Human growth hormone is expensive, available by prescription only, and in cases of genuine deficiency, has been shown to give important health benefits when taken under a doctor's supervision. However, unsupervised use of any hormone supplement can lead to health problems.

Keep in mind that although these findings may give new insight into the treatment of fibromyalgia, much research remains to be done. Although scientists are hopeful about this connection, it will be some time before new treatments will result.

Other Medical Modalities for Treating Pain

LOCAL INJECTIONS

A local anesthetic combined with a low dose of a cortisone derivative can give temporary relief when there are painful trigger points. Within a few days, there is often relief of pain from the localized trigger point and surrounding areas, with relief often lasting weeks at a time. This treatment is especially good when there are one or two trigger points causing major pain and limited movement. Also, if there is improvement in many areas but one or two painful areas remain, then local injection can be very helpful.

There are usually no serious side effects, and there should be no significant problems from an occasional local injection of these areas of tissue pain. This cortisone dose should have little effect on the rest of the patient's body.

OTHER INJECTIONS FOR PAIN

There are several types of injections available other than those used on trigger points. Injections around the spine in specific areas (epidural injections, facet joint injections, and nerve block) using a local anesthetic and a cortisone derivative may give pain relief that lasts for weeks or months. If this has positive results, the injections may be repeated after several months. Sometimes, stopping the pain temporarily may have a lasting effect on the chronic pain.

ULTRASOUND

Ultrasound uses sound waves that are applied to the muscles, tendons, and other soft tissues of the back. This may help relaxation, decrease inflammation, and improve pain in tender points. It is more commonly used for acute back pain and other similar situations than for chronic pain. It can be done properly by your physical therapist and continued if it gives relief.

TENS

Transcutaneous Electrical Nerve Stimulation (TENS) uses electrical stimulation for pain relief from many different causes. Electrical impulses sent to certain nerves block the messages of pain being sent by other nerves from the painful area. These impulses might also cause the body to release *endorphins,* which are natural pain relievers produced by the body.

The person wears a unit, a stimulator and battery, usually on a belt. Electrical wires from the stimulator attach to electrodes held by adhesive, usually a patch, on the skin. The electrodes are placed in the area of pain but may need to be tried at different locations to get the best relief.

The TENS unit can be used continuously or only as needed for the pain. Usually there will be a trial of about one month to see the effect on pain.

LONG-TERM NARCOTIC INJECTION

In unusual cases of some chronic pain, surgery can be used to insert a catheter for long-term use of drugs, such as narcotics, for pain control. A device called a *port* is installed, usually on the abdomen, which allows injections of medication as often as needed. A pump can also be installed through surgery to allow medication (such as morphine) to be delivered continuously for long-term pain relief.

COMPREHENSIVE PAIN CLINIC

As discussed in chapter 9, a comprehensive pain clinic may be useful, but only after you have tried the 7-Step Treatment Program and are still living with pain each day.

Read the criteria for finding a qualified pain clinic on pages 176 to 179, and with your doctor's consultation, choose one that best suits your particular needs.

Combining Other Treatment with Medications

In our clinic, we find that a combination of heat and exercise, along with one of the antidepressant medications and the most effective nonsteroidal anti-inflammatory drug, gives the best relief in the deep muscle pain. I will tell you up front that choosing the medications does require some trial and error. However, it is important that you patiently try the available medications in each group to be sure you have the best chance for success in pain control and increased activity.

Minimize Food and Drug Interactions

There are preventive measures you can take to ensure the least possible interaction between food and the drugs you take. Some medications must be taken immediately following a meal; others must be taken on an empty stomach. Some medications cannot be mixed with alcohol or the end result can be deadly. If you drink alcohol with an antidepressant, for example, the results can be excessive intoxication. Alcohol taken with a muscle relaxant depresses brain activity, and alcohol with a hypnotic/sedative (sleeping pill) causes oversedation and can even be fatal. Carefully follow your pharmacist's instructions on each prescription and over-the-counter medication you take, and be sure to contact your physician if you have any questions concerning medication and possible reactions.

COMMON FOOD AND DRUG INTERACTIONS

	Take on empty stomach	Take with food	Avoid alcohol	May increase appetite for carbs	Watch for stomach upset	Causes dry mouth
Acetaminophen (Tylenol)	✿		✿			
Aspirin (Many brands)		✿			✿	
Amitriptyline (Elavil)		✿	✿	✿		✿
Ibuprofen (Advil, Motrin)		✿	✿	✿		
Naproxen (Aleve)		✿	✿	✿		

Trial and Error to Wellness

In short, there is hope to treat fibromyalgia's symptoms. Although there is no quick fix, you can find success with treatment using a trial-and-error procedure. That is, you must work with your physician and try various medications and medical or complementary treatments to find the ones that will help. This will take some time as you sort through the options, but you will see greater benefits in the long run with symptom control, including pain management and less fatigue.

4

STEP 2:
EXERCISE DAILY FOR
MOBILITY AND ENERGY

Janet spoke of living with the symptoms of fibromyalgia for five years, traveling from doctor to doctor, complaining of widespread pain, tenderness at specific tender points, muscular weakness, and an overall flulike exhaustion. "I think most of them thought that I was this stereotypical hysterical female, but I knew differently. I knew that something was terribly wrong with me," she said.

This thirty-four-year-old mother and homemaker was an avid runner before she had children. "In college I used to run several miles each day before classes," she continued. "Then I started my career and family, and I never found time to exercise. Now I couldn't exercise if I wanted to."

This young woman is characteristic of so many patients, that is, most are aerobically unfit and not engaging in any regular exercise. Research has found that fibromyalgia patients are more than *75 to 80 percent below average in fitness* compared with age- and gender-matched subjects of the general population.

I have heard myriad reasons from patients as to why they avoid exercise, including:

> "How can I exercise? I can hardly walk to my car each morning."
> "Sure I'd exercise if only I had some energy."

"Exercise frightens me. What if it makes this disease worse?"

"I tried to walk around the block the other day, and it left me exhausted."

"There's no way this tired body can exercise. I can hardly make dinner."

"If I could ever sleep all night without tossing and turning, then maybe I'd feel like exercising."

"If you could cure me of fibromyalgia, I'd be glad to start exercising."

Exercise Is Essential for Muscle Strength and Flexibility

Both as a doctor and as someone who exercises daily, I know that a regular exercise program is essential to keep muscles strong and flexible, to control weight, and to stay active in other areas of life. Aerobic exercise particularly has also been shown to improve symptoms and restore muscle strength in patients with fibromyalgia. In fact, exercise and activity allow patients to have some control over the disease and the amount of pain they feel.

If you want to reduce your pain and get more energy, you will have to start exercising. Lou was the most resistant patient I'd ever treated when it came to moving around. Even though she had successfully followed the other steps in the treatment program, she refused to exercise.

"When I think of moving my legs and arms, all that comes to mind is pain, pain, and more pain," Lou said strongly. "And I'm sick and tired of living with pain."

It took three months to convince Lou that even though the pain wouldn't go away immediately, she would begin to notice a difference in her pain threshold within several weeks of starting her exercise program. And at her six-month visit, Lou found that exercise was the missing link in her treatment. Six months before, this fifty-two-year-old woman could hardly climb up onto the examining table. Now Lou was lifting her arms and stretching down to the floor—without pain.

In our clinic, we see patients who are able to see and feel great improvement with managing symptoms by maintaining a regular exercise program. Not only does exercise slow down the heart-racing adrenaline associated with stress, but those with fibromyalgia experience the added benefit of boosting levels of endorphins (proteins that reduce feelings of pain and induce euphoria), helping to relieve low-grade depression, and also helping them to receive restful sleep.

Exercise Boosts Serotonin Levels

Serotonin is a neurotransmitter in the brain that scientists have found to be related to fibromyalgia. (Neurotransmitters are chemicals that send specific messages from one brain cell to another.) While only a small percentage of all serotonin (1 to 2 percent) is located in the brain, this neurotransmitter is believed to play a vital role in mediating moods.

Studies have found that too much stress can lead to permanently low levels of serotonin, which can create aggression. When serotonin levels are increased in the brain, it is associated with a calming, anxiety-reducing effect, and in some cases, with drowsiness. Also, a stable serotonin level in the brain is associated with a positive mood state or feeling good over a period of time. Lack of exercise and inactivity can aggravate low serotonin levels.

It also appears that women may have a greater sensitivity to the changes in this brain chemical. Mood swings during the menstrual cycle, menopause, or following the birth of a child may be induced by the action of hormones on neurotransmitters.

Various factors can have a positive effect on serotonin levels, including sunlight, certain carbohydrate foods, some hormones, and exercise. Not only does exercise act as nature's

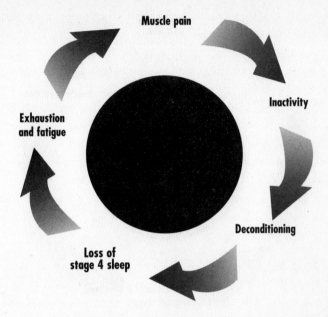

Figure 4.1. The cycle of inactivity.

tranquilizer, helping to boost serotonin levels in the brain, but studies have shown that exercise also triggers the release of epinephrine and norepinephrine, which are known to boost alertness. For those who feel stressed-out frequently, exercise will help to desensitize your body to stress.

Before starting an exercise program, most patients experience a cycle of inactivity that usually begins with muscle pain and leads to inactivity, poor physical conditioning, and disrupted stage 4 (delta) sleep. This vicious cycle can be halted with increased exercise and fitness.

Exercise: Safe and Necessary

Until recently, many researchers felt that exercise might exacerbate fibromyalgia's symptoms or accelerate the disease; thus, physicians encouraged patients to seek rest, not activity.

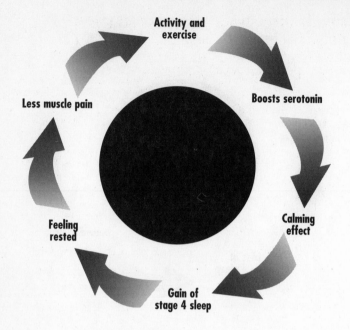

Figure 4.2. The cycle of activity.

But more recent scientific tests are conclusive in determining that, for most patients, range of motion, strengthening, and aerobic conditioning exercises are safe and necessary.

Most patients have a reduced quality of life, which can be the result of impaired endurance. Because of this, exercise is one of the first modes of treatment I encourage patients to undertake in order to reduce pain, improve endurance for physical activities, improve cardiovascular fitness, and cope with life's stressors, including their disease, in a more accepting manner. In fact, I have found that most patients can push themselves to exercise, even if they have not exercised for years and are in some pain.

If you are considering undertaking the recommended exercise program described in this book, I urge you to consult first with your physician to determine that it is safe to exercise.

BENEFITS OF REGULAR EXERCISE FOR FIBROMYALGIA PATIENTS

- Improves sense of well-being
- Strengthens bones
- Strengthens muscles
- Gives range of motion to painful muscles and joints
- Increases aerobic capacity
- Improves quality of sleep
- Stimulates growth hormone secretion
- Burns calories and makes weight control easier
- Increases cardiovascular health
- Reduces anxiety levels and depression
- Secretes endorphins or "happy hormones"
- Improves outlook on life
- Relieves stress associated with a chronic disease
- Increases energy
- Places the responsibility of healing in the hands of the patient

Different Types of Exercise

As you begin your exercise program, you will focus on three different types of exercise:

Range-of-motion or stretching exercises. These involve moving a joint as far as it will go (without pain) or through its full range of motion. The range-of-motion exercises or stretching will help you maintain flexibility in your muscle groups.

Endurance or conditioning exercises. When you increase your endurance threshold with cardiovascular forms of exercise, such as walking, biking, or swimming, you will not only strengthen your muscles, but also condition your body and build coordination and endurance.

Strengthening exercises. These exercises help to build strong muscles and tendons needed to support your joints. I recommend cautiously performing strength training using either resistance machines, resistance bands, or free weights (handheld weights that are not part of a machine).

Range-of-Motion or Stretching Exercises

Flexibility, the ability to move your joints through their full range of motion, is one of the key elements of fitness, along with cardiovascular endurance and muscle strength. Yet most patients have become inflexible because they have avoided exercise due to fatigue. This condition varies from one person to the next, as one patient may be flexible in her spine yet stiff in her shoulders. Another person may be able to bend down and touch the floor yet not be able to bend from side to side without pain and stiffness. Being flexible also helps protect you from joint injury, and the best way to get this protection is through stretching before activity or exercise.

More than anyone, sedentary people need the relief from muscle tension and stiffness that stretching provides. When done correctly, stretching feels good and is healing. Not only does a stretched muscle experience an increase in muscle tone, mobility, and greater circulation along with a marked decrease in pain, but also is less likely to be injured. Improper or excessive stretching, however, may actually increase the likelihood of injury—something you want to avoid with a chronic pain disease.

SEEK INSTRUCTION FROM A PHYSICAL THERAPIST

Because fibromyalgia's symptoms are physiologic in nature, you may want to seek instruction from a licensed physical therapist. These professionals have a background in anatomy and *kinesiology* (study of movement) allowing them to develop specific stretching and strengthening programs for your specific needs.

Physical therapy can enable you to regain control of your illness as you focus on lifestyle changes rather than on the chronic dysfunction. Proper posture, which your physical therapist will help you with, allows efficient muscle function, thus avoiding undue fatigue and pain. The slow stretching exercises on pages 202 to 212, performed *after* the application of moist heat, will improve muscle flexibility and reduce muscle tension.

Be sure that symptom relief modalities, such as heat and gentle massage, are only used for brief periods of time and in preparation for active exercise.

BEGIN A STRETCHING ROUTINE

Your stretching routine should be specific and include all the major muscle groups, including shoulders, hips, pelvis, buttocks, thighs, and calves.

Begin your stretching regime with five minutes of walking in place until your body warms up. This enables sore, tight muscles to loosen up. Then work at stretching one muscle at a time, holding your stretch for at least thirty to sixty seconds. A word of caution: Avoid overdoing this, as you don't want to add more damage to your aching muscles.

Although it is important to get to the point where you can do stretches daily, you must make a conscious effort to do the exercise correctly in order to obtain optimal benefit. It is better to do only a few stretches correctly than to hurry through them and risk injury.

Again, if stretching is done right, it should feel good. If you experience pain, check with your physician or physical therapist. The goal of stretching is to *decrease* pain and immobility, not increase it.

For more information about how to stretch properly, check with a physical therapist in your area. You can seek recommendations from your physician or contact the Private Practice Section, American Physical Therapy Association (see Resources, page 214).

Endurance or Conditioning Exercises

Recent studies have shown that aerobic fitness is a factor in regulating the altered sleep patterns characteristic of fibromyalgia. Tests have been done on patients, comparing aerobic exercise to range-of-motion or stretching exercise. Although both were found beneficial, patients who performed aerobic exercises regularly showed greater improvement in quality of sleep and trigger-point pain thresholds.

In our clinic, we find that some of the best types of conditioning exercises for patients are walking and water exercises. When performed regularly, these cardiovascular exercises can strengthen muscles and help to relieve depression. And then there's the added benefit of aerobic exercise: It not only challenges the heart and lungs, but by sustaining an elevated heart rate, it will enable you to burn fat and control your weight. Maintaining a normal weight is important for people with any type of chronic pain. It enables you to have more energy and relieves you of unnecessary pressure on painful muscles.

Again, your warm-up should include walking in place for several minutes along with stretching your muscles and joints in full range of motion.

CHECK YOUR PULSE

During exercise, it is important to take your pulse periodically. You can do this by placing your finger (not your thumb) on the artery on the side of your windpipe (your carotid pulse) or on the thumb side of the wrist. Slow your pace during your workout and count your pulse rate for ten seconds. Multiply this number by six to get your total pulse for one minute.

Your pulse rate should stay within your target heart range during exercise. This range can be found using the chart on page 81. Or, you can compute this yourself by subtracting your age from 220 and multiplying the number you get by 60 percent. This gives you the low end of your range. Now subtract your age from 220 and multiply this number by 80 percent to get the high end of your range. If your total pulse rate is higher than your target range, you should slow down. If the pulse rate is lower than the range, you may choose to work harder. Some inactive patients will find that their pulse rate will increase with very little exercise or activity.

ESTIMATED TARGET HEART RANGES FOR VARIOUS AGES DURING EXERCISE

Age	Low	High	Age	Low	High
20–21	120	162	54–55	102	132
22–25	114	156	56–57	96	132
26–27	114	156	58–59	96	126
28–29	114	156	60–62	96	126
30–35	114	150	63–65	96	126
36	108	150	66	90	126
37–44	108	144	67–70	90	120
45	108	138	71–74	90	120
46–51	102	138	75	90	114
52–53	102	132	76–78	84	114

The chart provides an estimate for the low and high end of your target heart rate. During exercise, find your pulse rate for one minute as directed. This total rate should fit within the recommended range for safe exercise.

START WITH WALKING

Walking may be the best all-around exercise for people with fibromyalgia. It can be done by almost anyone at any time and at any place . . . and it's free! I've seen patients improve their symptoms of pain, stiffness, and fatigue by simply adding fifteen to twenty minutes of walking to their daily routine. Because this low-impact form of exercise is less likely to cause an injury than running or aerobics, it is preferred by many as a safe way to become conditioned.

Beatrice, a forty-four-year-old woman who has lived with fibromyalgia for seven years, said that walking boosts her spirits, especially on days when pain and fatigue seem to overwhelm her. "I love to walk and hike in our neighborhood," she said. "On really bad days when my symptoms flair, I make myself walk anyway. I take a cane to give me added support and allow more time."

Not only will walking tone the muscles in your legs and upper body, but it will increase your metabolism and help with weight management. For women, walking offers a much needed bonus, as it increases bone density, which helps prevent a common disease of aging, *osteoporosis* (brittle bones).

You may wonder about those patients who can barely stand up, much less begin a walking program. In my experience, most people can start this program by making small goals. For example, if you have great pain during movement, begin by walking indoors from room to room for five minutes. As you progress in strength, walk around your house or apartment; then walk around your block. Your pace will depend on your capability and pain threshold, but by taking small steps, most people can achieve an adequate level of fitness. Remember, walking some is better than not walking at all.

Many prefer an indoor treadmill that can be used at home, so bad weather is no excuse, and it can be done anytime, day or night.

REFRESH WITH WATER EXERCISES

Perhaps more than any other conditioning exercise, my patients tell of enjoying water exercises the most. Forty-one-year-old Robert said that water exercise is almost as refreshing as a nap. "I can be having a rough day, feeling sorry for myself and aching all over, then I go over to the swimming pool at my apartment complex and get in the water. Something magical happens while exercising. In just minutes, I feel more optimistic and less pain. It works wonders for me and even helps me to sleep more soundly."

Numerous studies have been done recently on the benefits of water exercise to people with arthritic diseases. The findings are consistent with what Robert claims, that is, water exercise is a perfect no-impact activity that just about anyone can do without injury or stress to an aching joint. Most people report feeling better after a water exercise routine. Stretching or even walking in water is particularly comforting as the buoyancy of the water supports your body, putting less pressure on trigger points.

There are water vests and life jackets you can purchase that allow you to exercise in water without fear of going under. An aqua vest will place you in a near weightless position so you can stretch and strengthen muscles easily.

Most YMCA programs offer aquatic classes, teaching you the range-of-motion and aerobic exercises that can be done in water. Often, special classes are offered specifically for people with arthritis, and the trained instructors can assist you in designing a water exercise program for your specific fibromyalgia needs.

Strengthening Exercises

For those over the age of forty the muscle pain and weakness associated with fibromyalgia present an even greater problem. Studies show that muscle strength naturally levels off at mid-life. There is good news, though; resistance or weight training can offset this muscle decline and help build strength in aching muscles.

Studies have found that weight training brings about marked improvement for patients, although over the past decades, a greater emphasis has been placed on aerobics than weight training for pain relief. However, aerobics is a conditioning exercise for the heart and is not designed for developing muscle size. I have seen many patients become discouraged when, after weeks of aerobic exercise, they don't feel any lessening in deep muscle pain. That is why in order to strengthen your muscles, it is important to supplement your exercise routine.

COMMON MISCONCEPTIONS OF WEIGHT TRAINING

"I don't want to look like a football player," one petite woman said after we set her up with a qualified personal trainer to help with a resistance training program. Many people still associate weights with building bulky muscles, but this is not the case. Let's look at some of the common misconceptions of weight training.

1. Weight lifting is dangerous. False. If done with proper technique, lifting weights is a very safe way to tone the body.

2. If you stop, muscles will turn to fat. False. This is physiologically impossible. If you stop weight lifting, the muscles will lose size and tone, and any excess calories will be deposited as fat.

3. Women will get big muscles. False. Women produce less testosterone than men and build muscle size less rapidly. It takes years of hard work and proper diet to obtain large muscles.

4. Strength training means using heavy equipment. False. Resistance bands can be used as strength training. Other ways to strength-train include using isometrics, free weights, or even water-resistant exercises.

5. You must start with heavy weights. False. You should *not* begin with heavy weights. A good rule is to start with a weight you can easily lift ten times with the last two repetitions being increasingly difficult. For some people this is only one to two pounds; others can start at fifteen to twenty pounds, depending on their muscle strength. As your muscles gain strength and if there is no pain, increase the weights in one- to two-pound increments.

6. The theory "no pain, no gain" is true for strength training. False. If your muscles are very sore, do not use resistance training until you are relatively pain-free. Strength training may not be appropriate for every patient; check with your doctor for approval.

7. You will get high blood pressure. False. Weight training does not cause high blood pressure. Some people strain their body and hold their breath during a lift, which results in a temporary increase of blood pressure. However, holding your breath is *never recommended* during weight training.

8. You will become bulky and inflexible. False. It is important to supplement your weight training with a stretching routine to stay flexible.

9. Lifting weights helps you spot-reduce specific areas of your body. False. Exercise is not site-specific; you must exercise the total body to achieve maximum results.

10. The benefits are many. True. Increased strength, improved muscle tone, enhanced athletic performance, increased bone, tendon, and ligament strength, injury prevention, and improved body image are all benefits of weight training. For women, weight training can play a significant role in preventing osteoporosis, as bones need regular resistance to stay strong. And age is no factor with weight training; the muscles of older people can be responsive to training.

GETTING STARTED WITH WEIGHT TRAINING
As you plan your resistance program, you should lift at least two to three times per week, with at least forty-eight to seventy-two hours between sessions for muscles to recover. Select an exercise for each of the body parts: legs (calves,

quads, and hamstrings), abdomen, back, chest, shoulders, and arms (biceps and triceps).

One problem with weight training: Neglecting to exercise a body part can lead to imbalances in your body. Proper form is critical, whether you use free weights or machines. To ensure proper form and technique, it would be advantageous to use a qualified personal trainer the first few sessions. Your physician can help you find a trainer, if needed.

Initially, you should start out using very light weights or resistance of only one to two pounds, concentrating more on form. You can gradually add weight as long as proper form is maintained. Once you find a comfortable weight, you should stay with that weight for one to two sets of ten repetitions per body part, taking one to three minutes between sets to ensure a good quality workout.

TRY CIRCUIT TRAINING

Another way to weight-train is called circuit training. This is a group of machines that exercise all the body parts. You may be less likely to get injured using machines than using free weights. Free weights also can take months of practice before you become adept at sophisticated lifting techniques.

Heat or Ice?

All of the exercises described in this chapter will be much more effective and you will be more comfortable doing them if, before beginning, you take a warm shower for five to ten minutes to help you loosen up. You can even begin stretching while in the shower. After you complete the exercise program, take another warm shower if you have pain.

Some people feel more relief when they use ice packs instead of moist heat. A plastic bag or ice bag filled with ice can be applied to the painful area for about ten minutes. Don't place ice directly on your skin. Some patients get the most relief when they alternate treatments—moist heat then ice pack. Choose the combination that works best for you.

Remember—those who do their exercises regularly have a much higher chance of improving their symptoms. Do your exercises on good days and bad days, even when it is inconvenient. Once you are used to exercising, the time needed will be minimal and the rewards will be great. People frequently tell me that when they do their exercises they feel much better—and when they skip them, they feel worse. Exercises work!

Exercise Cautions for Fibromyalgia Patients

Although an ongoing, daily exercise program will help you to see the short-term results of increased mobility and decreased pain, it can take months to build strong muscles. You can make the muscles that support your aching joints stronger and more flexible, but it takes time.

It is important to set personal exercise goals as you begin the prevention plan. Your goal may be to exercise for five minutes each day for the first two weeks. Once you get in the habit of doing this, then increase this exercise goal by another five minutes until you reach the suggested fifteen to twenty minutes or more of conditioning exercises, four to five times a week. Be sure you include a warm-up (walking or light jogging in place) before you begin your workout, then move to stretching, conditioning, and a few minutes of cooldown, which can include walking around while stretching your muscles again.

5

STEP 3:
DE-STRESS YOUR LIFE

Doctor, I do apologize for being here, for I know you think I'm crazy." If I've heard this statement once, I've heard it hundreds of times. The varying, nonspecific symptoms of fibromyalgia, along with no scientific means to diagnose the disease, makes it is easy to feel as if the condition is imagined or in one's head. But research has shown again and again that fibromyalgia is not a psychiatric illness, even though millions of fibromyalgia patients have psychiatric symptoms, including depression, anxiety, and related disorders.

There is great speculation that stress or an inability to handle life's daily stressors may play an important part in the ebb and flow of fibromyalgia symptoms. Some researchers have tried to correlate high levels of stress with susceptibility to viral infection, whereas others have speculated that fibromyalgia could be viewed as "associated with dysregulation of the stress system."

If you are like many of my patients with fibromyalgia, perhaps you need to know how to de-stress your life so that these additional symptoms don't become a permanent fixture. Brenda, a middle-aged mother of teenage sons, tells of feeling nervous and having frequent panic attacks, especially when her fibromyalgia symptoms flair. But it may not be the fibromyalgia that is causing this excess anxiety; Brenda also tells of being "on call" for everyone in her family in addition to working part-time and caring for her aging parents.

Brenda's enslavement to pleasing those around her without thought of her own health and well-being is shared by many today, especially women. It can cause problems when you have a chronic disease and are faced with a new set of limitations. Fortunately, these limitations can be lessened, if you take active steps to get your life and priorities in order.

Is There a Fibromyalgia Personality?

Although in the past, some observations have described a stereotypical obsessive-compulsive, perfectionistic fibromyalgia personality, current studies do not support this observation. Using standard diagnostic criteria, researchers found that only 5 to 6 percent of fibromyalgia patients could be classified as having obsessive-compulsive disorder (OCD). Using psychological testing, these researchers found that approximately one-third of fibromyalgia patients are psychologically fragile, one-third have a chronic pain profile, and one-third are "normal."

It is important to understand that patients with fibromyalgia will always score high on the hypochondriasis and hysteria scales of these tests, since such scales are scored by summing the patient's physical complaints. It makes sense that if a well person were in constant pain and could not achieve restful sleep because of fibromyalgia, her complaints might also be magnified and appear to be psychological in nature.

While there is still some controversy regarding fibromyalgia and psychological problems, I have seen that when patients reduce stress in their lives, they also experience a reduction in depression, anxiety, and fatigue, as sleep becomes more restful. Because they feel more in control, the symptoms that were once immobilizing subside and quality of life is realized.

The Mind/Body Interplay

In simplest terms, stress is a response of the body to any demand. It is a biological phenomenon that affects both the central and autonomic nervous systems, as well as the endocrine and immune systems. And it is a key contributing factor to illness, including heart disease, depression, anxiety disorders, asthma and allergy, cancer, and even fibromyalgia.

While there is still some controversy regarding the role of stress in fibromyalgia, there are theories that suggest that it is the annoying daily hassles, not major life stressors, that greatly affect these patients and their symptoms. Especially when coupled with low levels of support from family, friends, coworkers, and even personal physicians, psychological stress may increase the patient's reaction to pain and escalate the chances that pain will occupy her attention. Some theorize that those with fibromyalgia experience higher levels of life stress and lower levels of social support than do healthy individuals.

Evaluate Your Stress Level

How often do you feel stressed? Some patients tell of feeling too much stress during the time when their symptoms flare. On the other hand, many fibromyalgia patients admit that they feel stressed every minute of every day. A recent survey found that 16 percent of those questioned felt stressed "all the time" and could not seem to relax, not even for a minute, while 52 percent of those questioned felt stressed "most of the time."

Every week an estimated 95 million Americans suffer a stress-related problem and take medication for their aches and pains. There are estimates that as much as 80 percent of all illness is stress-related, and 85 percent of all industrial accidents are linked to personal worker behavior that includes adaptation to stress. In new data from a study done by the Massachusetts Institute of Technology Analysis Group, researchers estimate that depression, which can be triggered by ongoing stress, costs American business $43.7 billion a year—as much as heart disease.

Study after study indicates that stress is skyrocketing, so you'd better fasten your seat belt, because there is no indication that stress will level off anytime soon. In fact, many people report that they are *more stressed* now than five or ten years ago. As Kim, a thirty-eight-year-old high school English teacher, said, "I get high anxiety just lying in bed thinking about what I have to do at school that day. Imagine how I feel at the end of my day!"

You don't have to imagine how Kim feels because you've probably been there. You know how stress makes your fibromyalgia symptoms worsen. Yet have you identified the areas in your life that are harried, hurried, and out of control?

Check each of the following problems or life interruptions that may negatively affect your body, and then use the suggestions in this chapter to make positive lifestyle changes.

___ too little sleep
___ too much sleep
___ negative attitude
___ hostility
___ depression
___ repressed feelings
___ sense of worthlessness
___ inability to communicate
___ poor diet
___ very little exercise
___ loneliness
___ recent job loss or lack of employment
___ job dissatisfaction
___ recent death of a loved one
___ caregiving to a chronically ill person

__ marital separation and/or divorce
__ exposure to environmental pollutants
__ smoking
__ heavy alcohol use
__ long-term medication usage

Because stress can show itself through a wide variety of physical changes and emotional responses in fibromyalgia, it is important to identify what causes these feelings. Stress symptoms vary greatly from one person to the next, and learning to identify the ways in which your body and mind show stress is an important step in treating and managing this disease.

THE SYMPTOMS OF STRESS
Anger
Anxiety
Back pain
Body aches and pains
Boredom
Bossiness
Change in bowel or bladder habits
Compulsive eating or gum chewing
Constant worrying
Crying
Dizziness
Dry mouth
Feeling of doom
Forgetfulness
Headaches and other aches
Inability to make decisions
Increased usage of drugs, alcohol, or cigarettes
Indigestion
Lack of creativity
Light-headedness
Loneliness
Loss of sense of humor

Memory loss
Palpitations
Racing heart
Restlessness
Ringing in ears
Sleep problems
Sweaty palms
Teeth grinding
Unhappiness

Not All Stress Is Harmful

Stress can be viewed as positive or negative, and the way we interpret the stress creates differences in our personal responses. In the past decade, research in the field of psychoneuroimmunology (PNI) has shown that life's stressors can produce the same initial physical response of adrenaline rush whether the stress is perceived as positive or negative. For example, you may cringe at the thought of skydiving, whereas your best friend would push to be first in line. Receiving an award and giving an acceptance speech might be considered exciting for one person, whereas even the thought of being in the spotlight might make another person visibly ill.

This observation also applies to those with fibromyalgia. I've had some patients who wake up anxious about what lies ahead of them, even when their day does not appear to be stressful. Louise told of how she would lie awake at night and anticipate how horrible she was going to feel the next day. "When the alarm goes off, I feel like crying. I'm tired from lack of sleep, my body aches, and I dread starting a new day," she said.

Yet other patients see each day as an opportunity, no matter what their pain or fatigue threshold is at that particular time. Raymond, a forty-one-year-old tax attorney, was diagnosed with fibromyalgia three years ago, yet he is certainly not waiting for this disease to take over his life. "I've got too much to do," Raymond said. "I've revamped my schedule to rest throughout the day, but other than that, I still do the very activities that I want to. I cannot imagine giving in to the pain and fatigue."

Both good and bad stress can affect fibromyalgia. The roles of perceived stress and psychological factors are controversial in fibromyalgia studies. Many reports show that patients report a heightened awareness of symptoms when facing stress, whether good or bad.

Good stress, or eustress.　Positive stress, or *eustress*, still signals the fight-or-flight response as does negative stress, but this adrenaline high usually gives us the energy to enjoy the moment. Positive stressors, such as a promotion or buying a new home, have been linked with increased productivity, happiness, and longevity. Yet for the person with a chronic disease, such as fibromyalgia, these positive events can also be interpreted in a negative manner. As one new grandmother told me, "Just thinking about traveling to take care of my new grandbaby makes me anxious and fatigued."

Bad stress, or distress.　Negative stress, or *distress*, also signals adrenaline to rush through your body, but it is this type of stress that puts you into the full-blown stress response and if continuous can lead to loss of productivity, burnout, and health problems, including a higher risk of getting diseases. For people with fibromyalgia, negative stressors, such as losing one's job or the illness of a loved one, can make symptoms that were controlled become active once again.

Stress and Fibromyalgia

The following list will give you an idea of what can add to your stress level each day:

THE STRESS IN YOUR LIFE

Waiting in long lines of traffic

Not being able to relax

Having fear of rejection from family and friends

Not getting recognized for abilities at work or home

Coping with too much noise at home or work

Going shopping and having to make choices

Having an overall dull feeling

Having to attend a party with friends

Not being able to express self

Not getting enough sleep

Meeting with the boss about a raise

Waking up feeling tired each day

Getting too much sleep and still feeling tired

Going out to dinner with family and friends

Overall tired feeling all day long

Annoying people

Being the guest of honor at a party

Misplacing or losing things

Going shopping with friends

Inability to concentrate at work or at home

Fear of confrontation with coworkers or family members

Entertaining friends at home

Inability to get close to coworkers or friends

Problems filling out forms

Preparing for the holidays

Dislike of preparing meals each day

Raising active children

Redecorating the house

Receiving a compliment from the boss

Having concerns about health and fibromyalgia

Vacation with family
Getting the yard work completed
Having no energy to do housework
Not having enough money to make ends meet
Too many medical bills, and the insurance won't cover all
    of them
Having to wait in line anywhere
Having to wait to see a doctor
Having a doctor not believe that the symptoms are real
Sexual problems with mate
Marital problems
Physical reaction to weather changes
Not enough energy to keep up in life
Declining physical abilities

After perusing the list, you may wonder why there are no major stressors listed, such as death of a loved one. If what current research indicates is true, patients with fibromyalgia are more stressed with daily hassles than they are with major life intrusions. In other words, waiting in a line of traffic or wondering how you are going to do your housework with all the pain and fatigue may cause you more apparent stress than a sudden crisis.

However, whatever your problems with fibromyalgia, too much stress does not have to be one of them. You can learn to manage your reaction to stress just as you do other areas of your life.

Melding the Body and Mind

Not only have scientists explored how stress may weaken the immune system, making us susceptible to diseases, they are also discovering how to meld the body and mind with psychological techniques—techniques that you can easily incorporate into your daily routine to reduce the threat to your immune system and well-being.

The key to reducing the stress that accompanies fibromyalgia lies in recognizing the signs and taking active steps to reduce these before the stress further injures your health and self-esteem. It is not difficult to start the stress-reduction program given in this chapter and incorporate it into your daily lifestyle.

Evaluate Your Commitments

BUDGET YOUR TIME
Do you find that there is never enough time in the day? Setting priorities and budgeting your time each day is the first step in gaining balance in your life, thus eliminating needless stress and anxiety. You can begin to do this by making a list of all of your commitments—family, work, community involvement, friends—and eliminating those commitments that are not absolutely necessary. Especially when you live with chronic pain and fatigue, you must allow for times during the day when you are not at your peak performance. This means not complicating your life with a list of activities and commitments that are just not important.

MAKE "TO DO" LISTS DAILY
Write down tasks that face you each day. As you schedule your day, budget ample time to get your work completed by calculating how long it will take to finish each project—then add on an extra fifteen to thirty minutes, to allow yourself to go at a moderate speed instead of in high gear. This will give you leeway, especially on days when pain and fatigue might hold you back from optimum performance.

If you find that you have more tasks scheduled than time available, rewrite your list and prioritize the projects that *must* be done; put the less important projects or activities at the bottom of the list. These can always wait until another day, or you can delegate them to others. Sharing the load is crucial as you learn to balance your day, doing what your body will let you do without excessive pain and fatigue.

Some people prefer to make their To Do lists each morning, while others find that doing it the night before relieves their minds and enables them to sleep soundly.

SCHEDULE YOUR DAY FOR PEAK EFFICIENCY

For those of you who work, staying employed is obviously a major commitment; but working late into the evening hours or seven days a week is something you can—and must—change.

Some people find that stimulation during late afternoon and evening hours makes it even more difficult to experience restful sleep; if you fall into this category, you may want to exclude evening activities. If mornings are your worst time with pain and fatigue, then plan your day around this and make your main commitments, such as business meetings or shopping, during midday or afternoon.

ACCEPT YOUR LIMITATIONS

When Katrina came to see me, she was at the brink of a divorce from her husband of nineteen years. "This disease has ruined my life. Not only have I lost my health, but my marriage is almost over." Through some intense counseling and a greater understanding of fibromyalgia, Katrina and her husband have worked through their marital problems. But first, she had to accept her limitations. Instead of denying the disease's existence and feeling anger and resentment for its symptoms, Katrina has come to accept it as a new part of her life, realizing that it is not terminal and learning to work around the symptoms to do the very things she enjoys.

Many of the fibromyalgia patients I've treated tell of always trying to achieve the best in whatever they do, and researchers are finding that perfectionism may be an identifying factor for those with this disease. A constant push for perfection can cause undue stress, which results in hazards to mental and physical well-being. Make sure that in all you do, the amount of time you put into the activity or job is well worth the end result. If it isn't, back off and let go of the perfectionistic attitude.

Which of the following perfectionistic beliefs motivate you each day?

- I must achieve my best, no matter how badly I feel.
- I cannot accept anything but perfection in all I do, or I criticize myself harshly.
- No matter how hard I try, I never feel like I've done enough or given enough.
- I would rather work at being perfect than spend pleasurable time with family and friends.

To reduce stress associated with fibromyalgia, you must realize that as a human being you are imperfect, even though you are endeavoring to become something more than you are now. Accepting this tension, you can begin to make some changes in your expectations of yourself. These changes can help you relax so that you can enjoy your life and experience a greater sense of well-being.

IDENTIFY YOUR PERSONAL STRESS REACTION

The initial impact of fibromyalgia on someone is always one of increased reactivity. This means that normally you may be able to handle a large workload, but now that you suffer with symptoms like constant fatigue, general feelings of anxiety or sadness, and muscle aches, any extra stress will put you in reactive gear. When we are in reactive gear, we are driven impulsively by our emotions and how we feel. Not only does reactive gear make us feel vulnerable, it can affect our relationships at home and on the job in a negative manner.

Determine how your body responds to additional stress now that you have been diagnosed with fibromyalgia. What are your stress warning signs as shown on pages 91 to 93? By knowing your own specific stress reactions, you can learn to listen to your body before the stress immobilizes you.

IDENTIFY AND REMOVE STRESS

The main strategy in dealing with stress is to identify and remove or reduce the source. If you react to the stress of being overworked, learn to delegate at your office or at home. If your stress is from overextending yourself with outside commitments, rethink how to modify your priorities and put this plan into action. If your stress stems from the fear of going to bed each night knowing that you are going to toss and turn, try to improve this by using the information in chapter 7 to ensure sounder sleep. If your stress is from facing each day knowing that you may have pain and fatigue, plan ahead the night before. For example, if you set out your clothes and get up thirty minutes earlier, you can move slowly without the necessity of hurrying.

As you seek to minimize stress, ask yourself the following:

- What stressors can I eliminate in my life?
- What stressors can I avoid?
- How can I reduce their intensity or manage them?
- What strategies do I need to use to make these changes?

MAKE JOB-SITE MODIFICATIONS

Fibromyalgia patients who are able to work outside the home tell of experiencing great stress on the job. Some tell of fearing they may be let go as healthier and more qualified workers enter the job force, whereas others are concerned that they are not able to perform the way they used to. Employers also tell of being concerned with the output of chronically ill patients, citing reduced productivity, increased absenteeism, poor work quality, and increased rates of on-the-job accidents.

To continue to be a productive employee, you need to stay mentally and physically able to handle your job responsibilities. You may need to allow more time during the day to get your responsibilities completed. Elizabeth told of talking with her employer about her illness and working out a plan that would benefit both. "I realized that I became very tired during midday," she said. "At that time, I was of no use to anyone, so with my boss's consent, I mapped out a plan to get my work completed on these bad days by taking a two-hour lunch break to nap, then staying a bit later to finish my reports. It has worked for both of us."

Other job-site modifications might involve taking work home on days when you feel fatigued or working on a Saturday morning so you can take extra long lunch breaks during the week to rest. Whatever you do, avoid procrastination. This may give you a break initially, but when it comes time for the work to be completed, you will feel more stress than ever. It has been said that procrastinators are perfectionists just waiting for that perfect time to do their work. Remember, there is no perfect time! Budget your time, follow your daily To Do lists, and limit your outside commitments on workdays.

Other steps for modifying work stress include:

- Ask for help from coworkers on days when pain and fatigue are overwhelming. Pay them back with your assistance on days when you feel better.
- Take periodic breaks to avoid getting overtired or stressed during busy workdays.
- Listen to music during your workday if you can to help keep stress levels low (see chapter 6 for benefits of music therapy).

Coping with work stress requires that you keep things in perspective. Again, this means that you must seek a balance between self, family, community, and work. This will help you maintain a support network to keep you centered and enable you to have strength to get through the day—even when symptoms flair.

INCREASE COMMUNICATION SKILLS

With a chronic disease like fibromyalgia, communication is the most important tool you have to decrease conflict with family, friends, and coworkers, especially when you feel anger or resentment from having unending pain and fatigue. Preoccupation with your illness causes a tremendous amount of distracting mental activity that can hinder productive communication. If you are feeling overwhelmed by the stress of fibromyalgia, you may find it necessary to have psychological counseling to help you develop appropriate and functional communication strategies to deal with your disease and its effect on your life.

Learn to say "no." Failing to set limits or say no to too many demands will put you in overload and add to your already rising stress level. Try to reach any decision that will involve a physical and mental commitment before you are put on the spot. It is much easier to say no to a persuasive friend when you have thought out the situation beforehand and have checked your calendar. Weigh the alternatives of making a new commitment, and include family members or friends in the discussion. Would another commitment prevent you from getting the rest, exercise, and relaxation you need to feel well? Would it take away from those priorities that are foremost on your list?

The desire to help others is commendable. But if being all things to all people is hindering your healing and making you feel resentful, tired, and depressed, it is time to take a firm stand. Say no—and mean it. You will feel physically and emotionally stronger if you make only those commitments that you can keep without undue stress.

Learn to remove yourself emotionally from stressful situations. Sometimes we magnify problems, making them seem far greater than they are. The stress reaction is triggered by our perception. When we imagine something to be a life-and-death situation, our bodies react as if we are in danger, even if no danger exists.

Work at tempering your emotions as problems come up throughout the day. Instead of every crisis being horrible, learn to view life's interruptions as inconvenient but tolerable. You will find that when you see life as something that you can easily handle, it will not overpower you when trouble hits.

KEEP A DAILY JOURNAL

Writing in a journal every day can lend itself to great self-inquiry and allow you to experience a higher plane of consciousness—with enhanced awareness, along with the practice of self-discipline.

With any chronic disease, patients often hide or are even unaware of intense feelings of resentment, anger, and loss. The intense self-inquiry process of keeping a journal can open the pathways to discover these destructive inner feelings and deepest concerns. Some patients can even identify a series of events that are associated with the beginning of fibromyalgia symptoms, offering a possible cause of how and when the symptoms began.

Keeping a journal can also assist you in tracking your muscle pain and fatigue and what the cause may be. For example, you may write in your journal that you are having great pain and feeling exhausted after working in your garden for several days. Months later, you can look back on this date and begin to see a pattern between the increase in your fibromyalgia symptoms and possible lifestyle triggers. Perhaps you find that you haven't slept well in days. Looking back over your journal will enable you to see any emotional or physical problems you may have had that contributed to the sleep problem.

ELIMINATE OR REDUCE CAFFEINE INTAKE

Caffeine is one of the few food products that mimics the stress response. Although a little caffeine may make you feel less tired on a bad morning when you've tossed and turned all night, too much can add to your already stressed emotional state, causing a short-term rise in blood pressure and increased heart rate and anxiety levels. Too much caffeine can greatly increase nervousness, which is a problem fibromyalgia patients do *not* need.

As you make plans to de-stress your life, try limiting your amount of caffeine intake, or better still, eliminate it altogether. Tea and chocolate drinks contain caffeine as well, plus ingredients like theophylline and theobromine, which also can stimulate the heart and central nervous system. Watch that chocolate candy bar you may eat, for it contains caffeine, too. I have found that there is no exact level of caffeine that is okay for everyone, so most patients choose to stop using it altogether.

FOODS HIGH IN CAFFEINE

Coffee, drip	5 oz. (90–115 mg)
Coffee, perk	5 oz. (60–125 mg)
Coffee, instant	5 oz. (60–80 mg)
Coffee, decaf	5 oz. (2–5 mg)
Tea, 5-min. steep	5 oz. (40–100 mg)
Tea, 3-min. steep	5 oz. (20–50 mg)
Hot cocoa	5 oz. (2–10 mg)
Cola soft drink	12 oz. (45 mg)
Chocolate bar	2 oz. (30 mg)

USE MIND/BODY TOOLS FOR RELAXATION

There is evidence that a variety of relaxation therapies, including meditation, prayer, music therapy, deep abdominal breathing, biofeedback, and visualization, are useful in reducing stress and stress-related illness.

When you meditate and experience the relaxation response, your body switches from the pumping "fight or flight" response to a calmer, more peaceful mood. Studies show that when you withdraw from problems and use mind/body tools for relaxation, you can produce alpha and theta waves consistent with serenity and happiness (see chapter 6).

Balance Your Life to Reduce Stress

In short, I know coping with the ongoing stress of fibromyalgia is not easy, but it is an important step in the treatment plan. High levels of stress can add to the wear-and-tear levels on your body and contribute to the pain, fatigue, and depression you already feel. This, in turn, can make it even more difficult to handle other problems that confront you each day.

As you begin to reduce stress in your life, work for an overall lifestyle balance. Make time to do the things you *want* to do, as well as the things you *have* to do. People with chronic diseases are faced with special demands that healthy people do not have. The task of coping with pain and fatigue each day makes it necessary to keep your priorities in order so you have the energy to reach your daily goals.

Remember, no matter what type of disease, all people with pain are stressed. Likewise, all people with fatigue are stressed. When you combine these two major symptoms in a disease like fibromyalgia, it makes it even more difficult to handle everyday issues, much less major life stressors that may arise. Although only you can get your life in control, do not feel as if you must do this alone. There are trained professionals ready to guide you and your family in a positive direction that will help you to understand and accept your illness and learn to live a quality life—doing the things you want to do—without restraint.

6

STEP 4:
TRY A COMPLEMENTARY
APPROACH TO RELIEF

Because fibromyalgia has no single mode of treatment but depends on specific lifestyle changes, you may discover that a complementary approach to healing is very effective in soothing the symptoms of pain, depression, and fatigue.

My patients tell of using safe forms of alternative or complementary treatment along with their regular medical regime. This treatment may include chiropractic, massage, acupuncture, and herbal or dietary supplements. Some find that a combination of complementary treatments—along with the medications, moist heat, and exercise—add a boost for healing, especially for chronic muscle pain that is unending.

Because the efficacy of many popular complementary forms of treatment has hardly been proven, it is important to weigh the pros and cons of using each, and evaluate the benefit to the disease. In my three clinics, it is only after discussing this individually with each patient that I offer my support and only if the following two criteria are met:

1. If the patient finds that the complementary treatment makes her feel better
2. If the complementary treatment does not hurt the patient in any way

Let's look at some of the most common forms of complementary treatment.

Massage

When you are very stressed and your muscles are tense, they
build up lactic acid. This makes the muscles even more tense.
Massage, a holistic philosophy for pain management, may help
to relieve this.

Studies released from the University of Miami School of
Medicine's Touch Research Center found that the benefits of
massage include heightened alertness, relief from depression
and anxiety, an increase in the number of natural "killer cells"
in the immune system, lower levels of the stress hormone
cortisol, and reduced difficulty in getting to sleep. Another
study reported that patients who received massage for pain-
related ailments took fewer narcotics or sedatives for the
pain—an important benefit for FMS patients. The patients
have reported a decreased heart rate and blood pressure and
even a reduced skin temperature.

Deep muscle massage affects the body as a whole. This
form of drugless therapy has been shown to increase circulation, give relief from musculoskeletal pain, act as a mind/body
form of stress release, increase flexibility, and increase mobility.

Massage therapy also:

- relieves muscle spasm and tension.
- relieves tension-related headaches and headaches associated with FMS.
- strengthens the immune system.
- reduces blood pressure.
- improves digestion.
- creates a calmer mind/body state.
- relaxes nervous system and reduces anxiety.

- releases endorphins (natural painkillers).
- can increase the levels of serotonin (a natural antidepressant).

There are several popular massage techniques:

1. General Swedish is the foundation for all other types of massage with particular attention paid to the back and chest. It helps to flush the tissue of lactic and uric acids and other metabolic wastes, as well as to improve circulation in the body without increasing the load on the heart.

2. Tapotement involves a percussion-type movement that includes four types of short, quick strikes made with the hands or fingertips:

Hacking: The massage therapist uses the heel or ulnar border of the hand on the muscles around nerve centers.
Tapping: Using fingertips, the therapist makes light to brisk movements.
Clapping: With the palms or the flat surfaces of the hands and fingers cupped, the therapist slaps the muscles.
Beating: The therapist performs this with a clenched hand on the buttocks and lower extremities.

3. Trigger point is a type of massage and pain-relief technique that helps to alleviate muscle spasms and cramping. This type has been found helpful for many with FMS. The therapist will locate active and latent trigger points, and mild to moderate pressure is applied for a short time (about seven to ten seconds). The muscles are then gently stretched to help the relaxation process.

4. Vibration is a type of massage where the therapist uses the heel of his or her right hand for vibration. The left hand is placed on top of the right hand for light compression.

There are other types of massage or bodywork techniques that may help deep muscle pain:

1. The Alexander Technique is a type of bodywork that is said to release painful muscle tension, improve posture, and reduce stress and fatigue.

2. Hellerwork is a therapy whereby the practitioner combines hands-on massage, movement, and dialogue to help you release accumulated stress and rigidity. Hellerwork is effective for temporary pain or tension relief.

3. Polarity therapy is a therapy where the practitioner uses gentle body manipulation and holding of pressure points to help restore natural energy flow. The practitioner will also educate you in exercise, nutrition, food combining, and maintaining a positive attitude to keep energy fields balanced.

4. Reiki is a type of bodywork based on the same energetic principles as tai chi and acupuncture. The Reiki healer rests her hands on various parts of your body in patterns that include the head, abdomen, legs, back, and feet. You may feel a sensation of warmth during this treatment.

5. Rolfing/Structural Integration is a therapy that promotes natural healing by realigning the body's underlying structure. The practitioner, or "rolfer," uses fingers, knuckles, and elbows to "sculpt" the client's body into correct alignment. This deep pressure applied by the rolfer helps to stretch the muscles and *fascia*, thick elastic connective tissue that envelops and supports muscles, tendons, and bones, making them more flexible.

6. Trager Method is a method of alternative healing that involves the use of movements, stretching, and pressure to help you give up muscular and mental tension and sink into a feeling of deep relaxation. Practitioners use movements such as gently rocking, swinging, stretching, and pressure to help you get into a very deep state of relaxation.

If you would like to find a qualified and licensed massage therapist, the American Massage Therapy Association provides a national referral service for qualified, professional massage therapists (see Resources, page 214).

Chinese Medicine

Chinese medicine is another alternative treatment many are turning to for fibromyalgia relief. This is a complete health system that has been used for more than five thousand years and is comprised of exercises, herbal medicine, massage, nutrition, and healthy living. Unlike Western medicine, which relies on aggressive and invasive action of surgery or modern drugs, Chinese medicine tries to diagnose disturbances of *qi*, or *vital energy*, in health and disease. Practitioners correct this disharmony in the body using acupressure, acupuncture, shiatsu, herbal medicine, Oriental massage, qigong, or tai chi.

According to proponents, traditional Chinese medicine has therapeutic value in the treatment of chronic hepatitis, rheumatoid arthritis, headaches, fibromyalgia, menstrual cramps, lower back and neck pain, substance abuse, hypertension, atopic eczema, immunologic disorders, and acquired immunodeficiency syndrome (AIDS). Although some scientific studies conclude that acupuncture and some herbs may have medicinal value, most Chinese therapies still need to be studied in the United States using the highest research criteria.

Acupressure is a well-known ancient form of physical therapy that was discovered before *acupuncture,* using the same points. This type of Chinese medicine therapy works by stimulating your body's main "trigger points" to release energy or unblock qi. Today, acupressure is mainly used to help alleviate pain associated with sinus pressure, leg cramps, headaches, temporomandibular joint disorder (TMJ), and carpal tunnel syndrome.

Acupuncture is a form of hyperstimulation for pain relief. There seems to be a close correlation between "tender points" and acupuncture sites used for pain control. A recent study published in the *British Medical Journal* compared two groups of patients with fibromyalgia. One group was treated with electroacupuncture and the other was given sham treatment during which acupuncture needles were inserted but somewhat less deeply, at a small distance from usually prescribed acupuncture sites, and with a slightly weaker electric current. There was improvement in actively treated patients in terms of duration of morning stiffness, overall pain, sleep quality, and overall assessment of disease compared with baseline. There was no significant improvement in the control group. These results were comparable to those reported for some medical treatments such as with the antidepressant drug Elavil, or amitriptyline (see page 53).

Western medicine research into the subject tells us that acupuncture brings relief through certain reflexes in the body that occur by way of the nervous system. That is to say by stimulating one portion of the body and using pathways of the nervous system, an effect is obtained in the same or another portion of the body. Additionally, it is believed that acupuncture causes the body to release endorphins that are the body's own pain-relieving chemicals.

Traditional Asian acupuncturists place the needles into specific acupuncture points along your body on lines known as meridians. Western doctors many times use the same points and may additionally use local trigger points, knotted areas in the muscle, which may be responsible for causing the localized or referred pain. Sometimes a slight electrical current is added (electroacupuncture). Acupuncture may therefore assist those with chronic, deep muscle pain, such as the case with fibromyalgia patients.

If you try acupuncture, with your doctor's approval, you need to go through a series of at least eight to ten treatments in order to ascertain whether it will be effective for you. You may not feel any relief, or you may feel extremely long-lasting relief. However, be sure that you go to a licensed practitioner who uses disposable needles.

Qigong is said to increase energy, decrease fatigue, and alleviate pain, all of which would be beneficial to fibromyalgia patients. Called the "mother of Chinese self-healing," qigong (pronounced chee-gong) is said to be one of the most powerful healing traditions ever developed in human history. When doing qigong, you will move into specific physical postures that help end tension throughout your body.

Initially, you may have to pay a practitioner to teach you qigong or sign up for a course at your local community center, but once you understand the positions, you can do this at any time at no cost. Those who regularly use qigong tell of needing less medication and faster healing. However, the postures or exercises should be done each morning to "build chi."

Shiatsu is another form of Asian therapy where the therapist focuses on relieving pain and helping your body rid itself of any toxins before they develop into illness. Firm, rhythmic pressure is applied for three to ten seconds on specific points. The practitioner will try to awaken the meridians, or healing channels, of the body. Scientifically, this applied pressure may stimulate your body's *endorphins* to produce a tranquilizing effect, or it may help by loosening up muscles and improving blood circulation.

Shiatsu may have great benefit to those with FMS, as it is said to help ease or eliminate back pain and sciatica, digestive problems, headaches, insomnia, leg and menstrual cramps, respiratory problems, and shoulder stiffness.

Tai chi may be the perfect exercise for arthritis sufferers and is used to help cope with tension and stress. It emphasizes complete relaxation and passive concentration without risk of injury. Some have even said that it is like "meditation in motion," with dramatic, flowing movements instead of forceful actions. The ultimate goal of tai chi is to bring the principles of yin and yang into natural harmony.

For those who find exercise painful, tai chi may enable you to slowly move your body in a full range of motion, building strength, while also receiving the benefit of stress reduction.

There are books on tai chi along with videos that you can purchase and use in the privacy of your home.

Chiropractic

Does chiropractic really work? It all depends on what it is used for. Chiropractic medicine comes closer to traditional Western medicine than the other forms described in this chapter. It is a drug-free approach to health that relies on manipulation of the spine and muscles.

Doctors of chiropractic are unique in that instead of treating the symptoms of a patient, they are primarily interested in treating the spinal bones when they lose their normal position and motion from stress, trauma, or other causes.

According to doctors of chiropractic, your nervous system controls all functions in your body; every cell in your body is supplied with nervous impulses. Messages must travel from your brain down your spinal cord, then out to nerves to the particular parts of the body, and then back to the spinal cord and back up to the brain. The theory is that abnormal positions of the spinal bones may interfere with these messages and oftentimes are the underlying cause of many health problems.

Doctors of chiropractic correct the abnormal positions of the spinal bones with what is called an adjustment or spinal manipulation. The doctor's hands or a specially designed instrument deliver a brief and accurate thrust. This adjustment involves the use of a specific force in a precise direction applied to a joint that is fixated, locked up, or not moving properly. Adjustments help return the bones to a more normal position or motion, relieving pain and ill health.

The chiropractic doctor will also recommend a program of rehabilitation for your spine. This phase of care is analogous to orthodontics. Goals are to stabilize and reduce joint involvement, rehabilitate muscle ligament tissue, and balance nerve impulses, helping you to regain maximum health.

Patients that do get significant relief from spinal manipulation find that it helps them to continue with their basic treatment plan of heat and exercises and allows them to resume a more normal lifestyle. Additionally, manipulation by a doctor of chiropractic, osteopathy, or other practitioner can be part of a total team approach to treatment with a neurologist, orthopedic surgeon, or rheumatologist to bring about the best total results for that patient.

Biofeedback

Biofeedback is based on the idea that when people are given information about their body's internal processes, they can use this information to learn to control those processes. This type of therapy has been shown to bring about improvement in the number of tender points, visual analogue pain, and morning stiffness in some fibromyalgia patients. In a study demonstrating the impact of biofeedback on FMS patients, fifteen patients who had a poor response to medication treatment were trained with biofeedback. After a fifteen-session electromyographic (EMG) biofeedback program, these patients improved in tender point count, pain rating, and morning stiffness.

Biofeedback requires you to be connected to a machine that informs you and your therapist when you are physically relaxing your body. With sensors placed over specific muscle sites, the therapist will read the tension in your muscles, the amount of sweat produced, or the measurement of finger temperature. Any one or all of these readings can let the trained biofeedback therapist know if you are learning to relax. When taught by a qualified licensed psychologist, with biofeedback the patient can control responses of the body, resulting in control of pain and stress.

The ultimate goal of biofeedback is to use this skill outside the therapist's office when you are facing real stressors. If learned successfully, electronic biofeedback can help you control your heart rate, blood pressure, and muscle tension when you are not hooked up to the machine. Some therapists recommend relaxation tapes that can be listened to at home to practice relaxation techniques.

Biofeedback has been found helpful in relieving temporomandibular joint dysfunction (TMJ), neck and shoulder pain, anxiety, irritable bowel syndrome (IBS), epilepsy, asthma, Raynaud's syndrome, hypertension, and incontinence. Some common types of biofeedback include:

Electromyographic (EMG) biofeedback. This type provides feedback on muscle tension and works well for patients with anxiety disorders or chronic pain.

Electrodermal (EDR) biofeedback. This type of biofeedback measures subtle changes in amounts of perspiration.

Thermal biofeedback. The temperature of the skin is measured and is used in teaching hand warming. This has been found to help relieve migraine headaches and can benefit those with Raynaud's disease.

Finger pulse biofeedback.　The finger pulse records heart rate and force and is useful for anxiety or cardiovascular symptoms.

Respiration feedback.　This type of biofeedback shows the rate, volume, rhythm, and location of each breath.

Hydrotherapy

Hydrotherapy works by stimulating your body's own healing force. Cold compresses reduce swelling by constricting blood vessels that help to control minor internal bleeding. Moist heating pads, whirlpools, or even a warm shower can reduce the soreness of aching or inflamed muscles. Even the simple act of running cool water over a wound can help rid it of dangerous bacteria and aid in healing.

The most common forms of hydrotherapy—ice and moist heat—are right at your fingertips. The next time you have unyielding muscle pain, use moist heat—a warm shower, a moist heating pad, a whirlpool spa, or even warm water running over the injury, sore muscle, or aching arthritic joint. For a new injury, apply the R.I.C.E. theory—Rest, Ice, Compression, and Elevation.

Detoxification

Detoxification is centuries old, going back to early biblical times when fasting was used as a method of spiritual cleansing. Avoidance of chemicals, from food or other sources, refined food, sugar, caffeine, alcohol, tobacco, and drugs is a safe way to detoxify your body and helps to minimize the toxic load.

Detoxification on a simple level makes practical sense, if you follow a healthful cleansing routine of exercise and sweat, fresh fruits and vegetables, increased liquids with more frequent urination, or more sleep when under stress. Yet the age-old theories behind colon cleansing or lengthy fasts are just that—ancient theories. In fact, many cleansing plans should not be done by expectant mothers, diabetics, and those who have chronic illnesses such as heart, kidney, or lung disease. Until research promotes these methods as safe and effective with substantial scientific evidence, stick to detox methods that you know to be safe.

Hypnotherapy

Hypnosis is another way to control the pain and stress that accompany fibromyalgia and has been highly endorsed by the American Psychiatric Association and the American Psychological Association. Although the word *hypnosis* comes from the Greek meaning "sleep," it is really an intense state of focused concentration.

In one controlled trial, hypnotherapy patients reported a better outcome with respect to their pain experience, fatigue on awakening, and sleep pattern as compared to patients receiving physical therapy.

Although this is not a "new" method of treatment, it is now being used in newer ways to improve the quality of life of chronic pain patients. With hypnosis, suggestions are made to the patient during a session that allow her to decrease the intensity of the pain, to move the pain to another area, or to try to build a feeling of separation from the pain.

Although this may sound too easy to work, hypnosis has been used successfully to help chronic pain in limited studies. I recommend that it be used to supplement other methods of pain control (such as exercises and medications).

If done correctly, this type of mind/body therapy can ideally produce a feeling of calm and improve a patient's confidence in handling the symptoms of fibromyalgia. Because hypnosis is not meant for everyone and may not work in every person, you should seek a qualified clinical psychologist or psychiatrist to help you decide if hypnosis would be helpful and safe for you.

Environmental Medicine

It makes sense that what we eat, breathe, wear, or sleep on can ultimately affect how we think, feel, act, and react. According to environmental medicine proponents, a wide range of toxic or harmful substances, including foods and chemicals found in the air, water, and food, can cause illness in the body. These environmental toxins, including processed foods and food additives, can tear down the body, resulting in poor emotional and psychological health.

Depending on your locale, exposure to toxins may affect your nervous system, lungs, and even your immune function. In some cases, it may have a bearing on your FMS. In fact, research studies support the use of environmental medicine for allergies, arthritis, asthma, chemical sensitivity, colitis, depression, panic attacks, reduced attention spans, eczema, fatigue, and hyperactivity. The treatment focuses on eliminating the environmental hazardous sources we can control. You may be told to modify your diet and to avoid such deleterious substances as strong shampoos, aerosol deodorants, cigarette smoke, exhaust fumes, organic solvents and pesticides, plastics, paints, perfumes and colognes, medications, gas used for cooking and heating, building materials, synthetic fibers, and certain clothing.

To see if the theory behind environmental medicine may help alleviate your symptoms, go through your home or office, and discover the problem areas. While environmental triggers vary, common triggers include aerosols, chemical fumes, cockroaches, cold air, dust, fresh paint, humid air, mold and mildew, perfume and scented products, pet dander, pollen, tobacco smoke, and wood smoke.

Removing those toxins you can control, and focusing on natural foods and household cleaning products, may help you to think clearer, avoid "fibro fog," and even regulate your moods.

Light Therapy

Light therapy is an up and coming alternative treatment that involves using natural or artificial light to cause physiological changes in the human body. Most recently, doctors are using light therapy to relieve the symptoms associated with seasonal affective disorder (SAD), a psychological problem that occurs with the change of seasons and less sunlight exposure. Those who have SAD feel depressed, fatigued, and may crave carbohydrates, as these carbohydrates boost levels of serotonin in the body.

Using specially made "light boxes," people are exposed to bright light and their bodies subsequently produce *serotonin*. With light therapy, women with PMS frequently report less depression, less moodiness, better sleep, and better concentration. Because of this boost of serotonin, light therapy may ease the depression associated with fibromyalgia. In fact, many mildly depressed individuals have seen improvement with just thirty minutes of bright light exposure; others may need up to two hours daily. This is consistent with the belief that light therapy helps people with winter depression because it makes up for light lost during shorter winter days.

Relaxation Therapies

As you've experienced, the daily stress of worrying about fibromyalgia and the limitations that accompany it can often put you in a state of emotional and mental overload.

The relaxation response, first described by Dr. Herbert Benson more than twenty years ago, is one of the most studied methods to reduce stress. Learning to induce the relaxation response at will can offer a real potential to reduce physical strain and emotional, negative thoughts—and increase your ability to self-manage stress.

Relaxation may be easy for some, but most people, even when they think they are relaxing, are not aware of the enormous muscle tension running throughout the body. However, by allowing time in your daily schedule to practice the suggested mind/body therapy and alternative treatment in this chapter, you can begin to get in touch with this muscle tension and learn how to end it—permanently.

Aromatherapy

This type of complementary "nose/mind" therapy involves the ancient art of using fragrances or essential and absolute oils and other substances for physical and psychological benefits. *Essential oil* is an extract or essence that's been distilled, usually by steam, from the seed, leaves, stem, flower, bark, root, or other parts of a plant, and an *absolute oil* is a very concentrated liquid taken from a plant and is extracted by alcohol. Essential oils are often diluted in a *carrier oil* such as sweet almond, grapeseed, olive, or canola oil before using with massage.

Each of the different aromas or oils has a specific healing power, whether to reduce stress, fight infection, increase productivity, or serve as an aphrodisiac. For example, lavender and spiced apples are said to increase the alpha wave activity in the back of the brain, which leads to relaxation. Increased beta activity in the front of the brain, on the other hand, shows greater alertness and is said to occur with the smell of jasmine or lemon. Some research has found chamomile essential oil to be an anti-inflammatory, and clove oil is antimicrobial.

Although it has been found that odors can change brain wave states, how do scientists explain this connection between odors and moods? Exactly how the scent/mood link works remains a mystery. Researchers do know that when aromatic molecules drift into the nose, they lock on to receptors there and create electrical impulses that travel up the olfactory nerves to the brain. One destination is the limbic system, where emotions and memory are processed. There is widespread agreement that these aromas help to increase the quality of sensory input for patients, thus reducing levels of stress.

Although there have been no controlled studies to date, claims rest on patients who say to have been healed or at least made to feel better with aromatherapy. Therefore, the answer as to whether scents can change one's mood and reduce stress could actually lie with each person. Sometimes fragrant oils are used in conjunction with therapeutic touch to ease the tension on the skin surface. These oils not only feel soothing to the touch, but also have scents that can evoke tranquillity.

There are two national professional organizations, the National Association for Holistic Aromatherapy and the American Alliance of Aromatherapy, along with a host of treatment centers across the nation specializing in this mind/body approach to healing and pain relief.

To use essential oils, try the following:

- Inhale the oil by adding 5 to 10 drops to steaming water or to a humidifier.
- Mix 1 teaspoon oil with 1 pint carrier oil, and use as a massage oil.
- Add 5 to 10 drops to warm bath water.

- Mix 5 drops with 1 cup warm water and mist into the air.
- Put 1 to 2 drops on top of the candle's melted wax, and inhale the warm scent.

ESSENTIAL OILS THAT RELIEVE STRESS

ESSENTIAL OIL	EFFECT ON THE BODY
Basil, rosemary, and lemon oil	Increases mental alertness
Lavender and chamomile	Relieves insomnia, PMS, and cramps
Sandalwood and geranium	Improves sex drive
Frankincense and marjoram	Soothes raw nerves
Jasmine and rose	Increases confidence
Lavender, vanilla, and chamomile	De-stresses
Basil, geranium, and orange oil	Combats depression
Peppermint and geranium	Boosts creativity
Orange, peppermint, and rosemary	Increases energy
Sandalwood and peppermint	Soothes upset stomach

Autogenics

Because the brain needs only a few reminders to calm down, autogenics teaches you to concentrate on raising the temperature of your hands and feet. Proponents claim that autogenics will give your heart a break from pumping so hard, open blood vessels, reduce breathing rate and pulse, and even lower blood pressure.

To do this relaxation technique, sit quietly, and put your left hand in your lap, palm up. Lay your right palm on top of your left palm, and clasp your fingers together. Concentrating on the feeling in your hands, *mindfully* (focus all attention on what you feel from moment to moment) work to raise the temperature of your hands for ten minutes. Then do the same with your feet. Counselors claim that if this is done correctly, you will feel "the heat" rise in both your hands and feet, indicating that your body is relaxing.

Laughter Therapy

Can a laugh a day keep FMS symptoms away? Maybe, according to many researchers. Laughter increases the activity of body cells that attack tumor cells and viruses. It helps to relieve anxiety, decreases stress-producing hormones, and increases immune system activity. In fact, many doctors are now prescribing "humor therapy" for chronically ill patients.

Norman Cousins was the first to promote laughter as an antidote to disease. While editor of the *Saturday Review,* Cousins was diagnosed with a serious connective tissue disease. After his doctors said that it was incurable, he was determined to get well.

During his journey to find a cure for his ailment, Cousins discovered that laughter actually affected his body chemistry in a positive, healing way. He filled his life with movies that made him laugh—"a real belly laugh." He then documented his account of the "miraculous recovery from laughter" in the book *Anatomy of an Illness as Perceived by the Patient.* As he recovered from his so-called incurable illness, Cousins went on to tell others of the miraculous power of laughter and about the resulting positive chemical changes in the body.

Today's scientists have found that laughing can produce a state of positive stress, or what is called *eustress.* In a study on laughter's effect on the immune system, researchers at Loma

Linda University in California showed a video of a comedian. Blood samples drawn during and after the video showed significant increases in various measures of immune function, particularly T cells and NK (natural killer) cells. Interestingly, the levels of the stress hormone cortisol, which suppress the immune system, were lower. The researchers concluded that laughter creates its own physiological state with positive changes in the immune system opposite those of negative stress or distress.

Meditation

Remember when transcendental meditation was thought to be a cult? Today meditation is recognized as a viable way to lower blood pressure, alleviate insomnia, and reduce chronic pain. This stress releaser seeks to integrate the mind, body, and spirit through intentionally focusing on the silent repetition of a focus word ("love"), sound ("om"), phrase ("peace heals"), or prayer ("thank you, God"). As thoughts intrude, you will continue to *mindfully* chant while facilitating the relaxation response.

This technique can guide you beyond the negative thoughts and agitations of the busy mind and allow you to become "unstuck" from your fear and other disturbing emotions.

Music Therapy

Music therapy has been proven to be an effective non-pharmacologic approach to assist in reducing fear, anxiety, stress, or grief in chronically ill patients. It is just beginning to make its mark as a way to treat pain and the stress that accompanies it, yet many are already reporting it as the best way to lower stress. Some researchers have found that in studies with chronic pain patients, the use of music can cause most patients to have a higher tolerance for pain.

Music therapy may sound too easy to work, but many of the sensations arising from music and pain are processed in the same areas of the brain. These areas are also responsible for coordinating our emotional responses. So, by focusing on and responding to music, perhaps we can block our bodies' response to pain. With this relaxation, we can decrease muscle tension and increase blood levels of endorphins. Although the level of pain does not change, having less tension and anxiety can make it tolerable.

For de-stressing, it is helpful to try music therapy in combination with another mind/body technique, such as deep abdominal breathing, progressive muscle relaxation, or guided imagery (visualization), as discussed in the following sections of this chapter.

If you employ music therapy as part of your treatment program, make sure that the pace of the music you choose is slightly slower than your heart rate, or approximately sixty beats a minute. This rhythm encourages your heart rate to slow down, and some studies of late have shown that this will also lower blood pressure. The works of Vivaldi and Chopin would fit this category, or you might try New Age music by artists such as George Winston with Windham Hill.

Deep Abdominal Breathing

Breathing can measure and alter your psychological state, making a stressful moment accelerate or diminish in intensity. Think about how your respiration quickens when you are fearful or in great pain, and how taking a deep, slow breath can have a calming effect, reducing both stress and levels of muscle pain.

Although we often take breathing for granted, this is one of the few activities of the body that we can consciously control. As you learn how to do deep abdominal breathing, you will gain control over a basic physiological function, helping to decrease the release of stress hormones and slow down your heart rate during stressful moments. Also, by adding oxygen to the blood, you can actually cause your body to release endorphins, the hormones that give a greater sense of well-being and contentment.

Lie on your back in a quiet room with no distractions. If necessary, take the phone off the hook so you are truly alone. Place your hands on your abdomen and take a slow, deliberate deep breath in through your nostrils. If your hands are rising, your abdomen is expanding and you are breathing correctly. If your hands do not rise, yet you see your chest rising, you are breathing incorrectly.

Inhale to a count of five, pause for three seconds, then exhale to a count of five. Start with ten repetitions of this exercise, and then increase to twenty-five, twice daily. Use this exercise any time you feel anxious or stressed. Some of my patients find it extremely helpful when they are experiencing great pain. As one patient, Laura, said, "When I have severe muscle pain, I use my breathing to go with the pain. Somehow, this takes my mind off the pain and lessens its severity."

Progressive Muscle Relaxation

Progressive muscle relaxation involves contracting and then relaxing all the different muscle groups in the body, beginning with head and neck and progressing down to the arms, chest, back, stomach, pelvis, legs, and feet. To do this exercise, you focus on each set of muscles, tense these muscles to the count of ten, and then release to the count of ten. Go slowly as you progress throughout your entire body, taking as long as you can. Get in touch with each part and feel the tension you are experiencing. Also, notice how it feels to be tension-free as you release the muscle.

Studies show that when you can create a strong mental image using this type of relaxation technique, you actually feel "removed" from cumbersome stress and negative emotions. This *mindfulness,* or focusing of attention, can also help you move beyond destructive habits as you become centered in a world of health and inner healing.

You can do this exercise with or without music, and it is important to perform it with deep abdominal breathing, focusing on your breath. Breathe in while tensing the muscles, and breathe out or exhale while relaxing them.

Guided Imagery Techniques

According to scientific tests, the mind cannot distinguish between fears, fantasies, and reality. Therefore, another effective mind/body technique for healing is guided imagery (also called visualization). This involves mentally seeing pictures of relaxing situations, such as a beach at sunset, a flowing mountain waterfall, or a brilliant mountain sunrise.

The power of your imagination is important in guided imagery, as you use sights, sounds, feelings, and smell to create a desired state in your mind. Used in combination with deep breathing, it produces long-term stress reduction. This technique has been used to improve the surveillance function of the immune system. Through guided imagery, you will reduce your anxiety level during stressful times and lower your heart rate and blood pressure. As you continuously visualize a positive healing image, you may significantly contribute to your own well-being.

If you have trouble imagining scenes and images, listen to sounds of waves or thunderstorms to trigger natural settings. Tapes can be purchased at any music store. Or, purchase postcards with peaceful, serene scenes on them, and keep these with you. Pull out your visualization cards when you feel your body tensing and you need to imagine being somewhere else where life is kinder and less threatening.

Homeopathic Medicine

Homeopathic remedies are regulated by the Food and Drug Administration (FDA). Proponents believe that this form of alternative medicine effectively treats allergic rhinitis, hay fever, migraine headaches, trauma, gastritis, allergic asthma, acute childhood diarrhea, fibromyalgia, and influenza. Yet lack of convincing scientific proof is one of the great problems with homeopathy's acceptance by conventional medical doctors. Critics believe that because the medications are so diluted, the only benefit received is placebo.

Nonetheless, a survey of 107 clinical trials published in the *British Medical Journal* (February 1991) showed that 80 percent were positive in favor of homeopathy. One landmark review published in the scientific journal *The Lancet* said that homeopathy was shown to be nearly two and a half times more effective than placebos in the treatment of such problems as arthritis, allergies, varicose veins, and gastrointestinal pain.

Some commonly used homeopathic remedies include:

Aconitum for PMS
Allium cepa for allergies and colds
Arnica for sore muscles, bruises, and sprains
Belladonna for PMS and menopausal symptoms
Bryonia for constipation and vaginal dryness
Chamomilla for earache and PMS
Cimicifuga for PMS, anxiety, and depression
Cocculus for depression and sleep deprivation
Colocynthis for menstrual cramps and irritability
Conium maculatum for breast tenderness and swelling
Gelsemium for headache
Ignatia amara for depression and sadness
Lachesis for PMS, headaches, pain, menopausal symptoms
Natrum muriatcum for menopausal symptoms

Nux vomica for diarrhea, hemorrhoids, and constipation
Sepia for PMS, menopausal symptoms, and depression

If you seek advice from a homeopathic practitioner, be sure
this person is a medical doctor. Ask where he or she has studied homeopathy and whether a certification exam was passed.
Licensing is required in only three states at this time, and
there are no formal guidelines or formal schools for homeopathy. It is also imperative that you check with your own physician before taking any unknown substance or supplement
because of the possibility of allergic reactions.

Herbal Therapy

Herbal and other plant-derived remedies have been estimated
by the World Health Organization (WHO) to be the most
frequently used therapies worldwide. Although precise levels
of use in the United States are unknown, in 1994, herbal
products accounted for sales of more than $1.6 billion, the
fastest-growing category in drugstores.

Pharmaceutical companies are very interested in herbal
therapy, and reports show that more than 25 percent of all
prescription drugs are derived from these wild medicinals,
including the flowers, leaves, bark, berries, and roots of plants.
Although there are a few herbs that are dangerous and should
never be ingested or put on your skin, most herbs are safe.

Keep in mind that if you do choose an herbal therapy, some
therapeutic agents derived from plants include pure chemical
entities available as prescription drugs (e.g., morphine). Plant-
derived remedies can contain chemicals with potent pharma-
cologic toxicologic properties.

The problem with trying to purchase herbs that are
"guaranteed safe" is that there is no proof that herbal therapies work other than word of mouth from consumers. The
reason for this is that in order to get FDA approval, the com-

pany marketing the drug must prove that it is safe and effective. Plants cannot be patented, so most companies call herbs "foods" and market them in this way.

Herbal remedies have been used for generations and can be put in tea or soup or taken in other forms. Certain remedies such as alfalfa or chamomile are more popular in some areas of this country than in others. Although some herbal therapies have not been shown to have a specific benefit for arthritis symptoms, some patients have used the following with good results for helping to obtain more restful sleep or for more energy.

HERBAL TREATMENTS

NAME OF HERB	COMMON USES
Blackcurrant seed oil	Suppresses inflammation and joint tissue injury.
Boswellia	Relieves inflammation.
Cayenne	Acts as a pain reliever. Relieves migraine or tension headaches. As a salve or ointment, relieves muscle pain.
Chamomile	Helps calm nervousness, anxiety, menstrual cramps, and upset stomach. May boost immune function.
Echinacea	Boosts the immune system and helps to prevent infections.
Feverfew	Inhibits inflammation and acts similarly to aspirin.

NAME OF HERB	COMMON USES
Ginger	Stimulates mucus-producing vagus nerve reflexes and has an antioxidant effect and an anti-inflammatory effect.
Ginkgo biloba	Improves concentration and memory, increases blood flow, and helps the symptoms of PMS. Helps with short-term memory loss and depression.
Ginseng	Increases energy and relieves stress.
Goldenseal	Soothes inflammation of the respiratory, digestive, and genitourinary tracts caused by allergy or infection.
Goto kola	As "brain food," promotes memory, alleviates mental fatigue, and normalizes blood pressure.
Hawthorn berries	Strengthens the muscles and nerves to the heart.

NAME OF HERB	COMMON USES
Hyssop	Regulates blood pressure and promotes circulation. Relieves hoarseness, lung congestion, and mucus buildup.
Gotu kola	Helps to improve mental ability and relieves stress.
Kava kava	Helps to fend off anxiety and nervous tension. Also has anti-inflammatory effect on the body.
Kelp	Provides energy and endurance, helps to relieve nervous tension, and promotes circulation to the brain.
Lavender	Relieves insomnia, depression, and headache.
Licorice	Promotes healthy adrenal glands and acts as a sexual stimulant.
Meadowsweet	Acts to reduce inflammation.
Milk thistle	Bolsters the immune system.
Myrrh	Cleans the colon and soothes digestive system upset.

NAME OF HERB	COMMON USES
Passionflower	Acts as a mild tranquilizer and eases insomnia, stress, and anxiety.
Pine bark	Stimulates circulation and helps reduce inflammation.
Psyllium	Helps to restore tone to the intestines and lubricates and heals irritated tissues.
Pycnogenol	Boosts serotonin in the body.
Saint-John's-wort	Relieves depression without the side effects of prescription antidepressants.
Slippery elm	Relieves sore throats and soothes mucous membranes.
Valerian	Acts as a sedative and helps to combat insomnia.

TAKE A CAUTIOUS APPROACH TO HERBAL THERAPY

If you want to try herbal therapy, it is important to consult with your physician. Many times you may pick up something at the grocery or health food store because of an advertised "quick cure" for pain and stiffness, but when it comes to self-medicating with herbs, my advice is usually "let the buyer beware." Always know what you are putting in your body and on your skin. When herbal therapies are not approved by the FDA, they can be combined with other ingredients that could actually make your condition worse. In other words, while most might help your symptoms, others can be deadly.

Some patients have taken products containing ephedra, thinking it might help boost alertness and energy. It's important to know that the FDA recently proposed cracking down on the marketing of ephedra products, citing about eight hundred injuries and at least seventeen deaths linked to the herbal stimulant. Among the proposals are limiting concentrations of the herb in any dietary supplement, requiring warning labels that its use can cause death, and banning claims that it can help people lose weight or build muscle. Some popular products containing ephedrine include "Herbal Ecstasy," "Ultimate Xphoria," and "Herbal Phen-Fen." It is also marketed as ma huang, Chinese ephedra, and epitonin.

Natural Dietary Supplements

Dietary supplements include a host of products that contain vitamins, minerals, herbs, and amino acids as well as natural enzymes, organ tissues, metabolites, extracts, or concentrates. Some alternative practitioners recommend the following natural remedies for prevention and treatment of disease. Most are available at drugstores, grocery stores, or health food stores.

Chromium picolate is a trace mineral important in helping cells break down sugar into energy for the body. Supplements can help to regulate blood sugar, fat, and carbohydrate metabolism. Uncontrolled blood sugar levels can contribute to weight gain, high cholesterol, and high blood pressure. Interestingly, chromium seems to normalize low blood sugar. A recent USDA study of 180 Type 2 diabetics in China documented "spectacular" results from taking 1,000 micrograms of chromium picolinate daily with nearly all of the subjects no longer having the classic signs of diabetes. For those with FMS, taking chromium may help in stabilizing mood swings and anxiety caused by fluctuations in blood sugar levels.

CLA (conjugated linoleic acid) is a fatty acid that is said to reduce fat by inhibiting the body's ability to store fats. It also has antioxidant properties, increases muscle tone, and improves food efficiency.

Coenzyme Q10 is a natural substance that improves heart and immune function. It is also an antioxidant that helps to lower cholesterol levels and reduces oxidative damage to blood vessels.

Essential fatty acids (EFAs) are not manufactured by the body, but these fats are essential to cardiovascular health and normal brain development. EFAs are available in oils containing omega-3 (fish oils) and omega-6 (linolenic and gamma-linolenic, or GLA, which are found in plant oils such as evening primrose, black currant, and borage).

Glucosamine and **chondroitin** are two substances that the human body produces to make cartilage. In supplement form, glucosamine comes from crab shells, and chondroitin comes from cow cartilage. Although scientific studies have yet to call these the "cure" for arthritis, in some studies of people with arthritis, the supplements were found to ease aches as well as over-the-counter painkillers, but more slowly. Although their long-term safety has never been established, they appear to have no side effects, and researchers do not know whether you must take the two supplements together or if one is effective taken by itself. If you have osteoarthritis along with fibromyalgia, this natural solution may help you.

Lecithin is commercially isolated from soybeans, corn, and eggs and may help with easing the memory glitches that happen with aging. Just two tablespoons of lecithin a day stimulates the body's output of choline, a brain chemical that is important in recall and memory.

Melatonin is a natural hormone secreted from the pineal gland in the brain. It has a major influence on the human body's inner clock, which governs the sleep-wake cycle and other biological functions (see pages 61 and 62).

Get the Best of Both Worlds

It is important to be open-minded as you consider alternative treatments for fibromyalgia. You don't want to miss a chance for good relief, but you also don't want to take unnecessary risks.

When patients come to me with a new remedy that is an alternative treatment, I ask them to consider the following:

- Is it approved by the U.S. Food and Drug Administration (FDA)?
- Does it have any known side effects?
- What is the expertise of the person administering the remedy?
- What has happened to similar treatments over the years?
- Will your health insurance company reimburse you?

Become your own expert. Beware of any treatment that promises quick and easy relief or a cure. If it sounds too good to be true, it probably is! You can receive more information on alternative treatments from the Arthritis Foundation and the Fibromyalgia Association (see Resources, page 215).

It is important to know when a substance may be dangerous to your health, and you should avoid any substance taken internally. For example, rattlesnake meat is a common remedy in some areas for many illnesses, including arthritis and back pain. But some forms of capsules containing rattlesnake meat have been shown to cause serious illness.

If an alternative treatment is proven harmless and won't delay proper medical evaluation and treatment, then it is acceptable to try. If you have questions about a new treatment, talk to your doctor and make sure it is safe to use. This can allow you to take advantage of newer treatments, but avoid those that may cause more harm than relief.

It is my experience that once patients have the diagnosis

of fibromyalgia and learn to live with it, they become the "experts" on their disease. Those who tell of feeling more energy and less pain have learned how to make lifestyle changes and use alternative and medical treatments in a complementary manner—in a way that enhances both health and well-being.

7

STEP 5:
END SLEEPLESS NIGHTS

Sleep deprivation was written all across Christina's face. Until she started treatment for fibromyalgia two years ago, this forty-seven-year-old woman lived for months with dark circles under her eyes from lack of restful sleep. Christina made it a point to be in bed by nine o'clock each night but then tossed and turned until sunrise and always felt too tired to go to work the next day.

Like Christina, the majority of fibromyalgia patients are fatigued, even after sleeping for ten hours at night. One woman said, "I go to bed tired and feel tired all night. I awaken tired, then I feel tired the next day."

Patients complain that no matter how long they sleep, it is never restful. Their sleep may be interrupted by frequent awakening, that is, becoming awake enough that they remember these times the next day. Even more common are awakenings that are not enough to remember but that definitely break up their deep sleep. Most patients tell of waking up day after day feeling exhausted. They feel more tired in the morning, and many have great difficulty in concentrating during the day, just as in other situations where sleep is disrupted.

Because obtaining restful sleep is a crucial problem with this disease, it is helpful to understand the characteristics of normal sleep and how this differs from the sleep experienced by fibromyalgia patients.

Understanding the Stages of Sleep

Studies have demonstrated that we have a built-in cycle of sleep-wake times along with many other cyclic variations in bodily functions, such as glandular secretions, body temperature, heart rate, blood pressure, and bronchial function. These intrinsic cycles are controlled by a group of nerve cells called a *circadian pacemaker*. This pacemaker is closely related to parts of the retina (in the back of the eye) and the hypothalamus in the brain.

The circadian cycle is actually twenty-five hours long. Since the cycle is longer than the twenty-four-hour day, some factor must serve to synchronize the body's pacemaker with the external clock time. These are cues from the environment called *zeitgebers* (from German, meaning "time-givers"). The most important and powerful one is light. The hormone most closely linked to the circadian system is melatonin, which is made by the pineal gland in another part of the brain. Melatonin has been shown to synchronize the sleep-wake cycle to twenty-four hours in some blind subjects who were otherwise unable to live on a twenty-four-hour day.

In adults, sleep is made up of distinct types or stages with specific characteristics defined by brain waves, eye movements, and muscle tension. The two broad categories of sleep include rapid eye movement sleep (REM) and nonrapid eye movement sleep (NREM). During REM sleep, there are small, variable-speed brain waves, rapid eye movements like those of eyes-open wakefulness, and absent muscle tension. It is during REM sleep that we have almost all of our dreams. (Arousals from this stage of sleep are usually associated with recall of vivid imagery.) In NREM sleep, there are four different stages—1, 2, 3, and 4—characterized by different combinations of brain waves, eye movements, and reduced but not absent muscle tension. In fibromyalgia, stages 3 and 4 NREM sleep are of most importance. These stages are defined by relatively large, slow brain waves (delta waves), absent eye movements, and reduced muscle tension. Other names for these stages are "slow-wave sleep" or "delta sleep."

About sixty years ago, it was recognized that sleep intensity is reflected by the amount of delta sleep. The depth of sleep is correlated with this stage, and it is from delta sleep that arousal is most difficult. Interestingly, growth hormone secretion is highest during delta sleep. Some researchers suggest this is important for growth and repair of body tissue.

The stages of sleep can be contrasted with the state of wakefulness. The wake state is associated with small, variable, but mostly rapid (seven to eleven cycles per second) brain waves called *alpha waves*. There are quick, alert eye movements along with variable, generally high tension in the muscles.

The stages of sleep are distributed through the normal sleep period in a particular pattern. Sleep onset usually is within five to twenty minutes of going to bed. After the start of sleep, there is a cycling through stages 1 to 4 approximately every forty-five to ninety minutes with REM sleep punctuating each cycle at about sixty- to ninety-minute intervals. Delta sleep occurs mostly in the first third of the night and makes up about 10 to 20 percent of total nocturnal sleep in normal young adults, whereas REM sleep takes place predominantly during the last third of the night's sleep.

The percentage of delta sleep is affected by age, amount of prior sleep, and various diseases. Delta sleep decreases with age and may be absent in healthy, elderly males. Sleep deprivation increases the rapidity of the onset of delta sleep and its portion of total sleep time.

Young children have particularly large proportions of delta sleep, which increases if they are sleep-deprived. This explains why it is frequently difficult to awaken children. Elderly people have smaller proportions of delta sleep, which is why they are easily aroused by environmental noise. Medical problems, such as obstructive sleep apnea, periodic leg movements during sleep, and fibromyalgia may affect quantity and quality of delta sleep. This in turn probably accounts in some measure for the feeling of fatigue experienced by people suffering from these maladies.

Fibromyalgia and Sleep

About twenty years ago, researchers in Toronto discovered that patients with fibromyalgia had NREM stages of sleep "contaminated" by an intercurrent alpha rhythm (like that of wakefulness). But whether the sleep disturbance caused the fibromyalgia symptoms or was secondary to the disease itself could not be determined.

This group of investigators went on to show that healthy subjects selectively deprived of delta sleep by being exposed to noise developed periods of delta sleep mixed with alpha waves. Interestingly, when deprived of delta sleep these people experienced some musculoskeletal discomfort and mood symptoms similar to those of the patients with fibromyalgia. These data suggested that the stage 4 sleep disturbance caused the appearance of the achiness or pain and mood symptoms.

However, it was felt that the effect of delta sleep disturbance on symptoms might be determined by examining the physical and psychological characteristics of the healthy subjects. Their subjects were younger than the patient population with fibromyalgia and free from illnesses and psychological problems, but they were not particularly physically fit. Yet they had the symptoms of fibromyalgia when put through the sleep-deprivation process. Their relatively sedentary lifestyle may have been significant, because most reports have pointed to the positive influence of exercise on delta sleep.

Sleep disturbances can be triggered in patients by physical or emotional trauma or by a metabolic or other medical problem. Poor sleep can lead to fatigue with resultant diminished exercise causing worsened physical fitness and the establishment of a vicious cycle of inactivity and sleep disturbance with physical and mood-related symptoms (see the Cycle of Inactivity on page 75). These problems could help lead to the development of fibromyalgia.

ACCURATE DIAGNOSIS IS ESSENTIAL FOR PROPER THERAPY

Many of the symptoms that fibromyalgia patients experience are shared by those with other sleep disorders. For example, some patients with obstructive sleep apnea, intermittent blockages of the upper airway at the back of the tongue, which occurs in 2 percent of women and 4 percent of men who are thirty to sixty years old, also complain of unrefreshing sleep and "hurting all over" upon arising in the morning. They also have a history of snoring and other symptoms, including morning headaches, dry mouth, and an increased tendency to doze off during the day. Some patients with sleep apnea have high blood pressure.

If your doctor suspects that your sleep disorder may have a different cause, he or she may recommend that you have a sleep study. Sleep studies, called *polysomnography*, include an *electroencephalogram* (EEG), which measures the electrical activity of the brain, as well as the monitoring of oxygen levels, movements of chest wall and abdomen, and nasal and oral airflow. A sleep study may show apnea (periods without breathing), manifested by absent airflow at nose and mouth in conjunction with ongoing respiratory muscle efforts shown by movement of chest wall and abdomen. An apnea may cause decreases in blood oxygen levels. Sleep is often interrupted at the end of the apnea by awakening.

This breaking up of continuous sleep is a major cause of daytime fatigue and sleepiness. Periodic leg movements during sleep, also known as nocturnal myoclonus, may also be associated with alpha intrusions and are a common cause of sleep interruptions. These sleep disorders require specific therapy.

It should be noted that certain drug therapy for fibromyalgia may worsen obstructive sleep apnea and actually exacerbate the patient's symptoms of fatigue and restless sleep.

The Problem of Insomnia

Because patients with fibromyalgia have a specific type of insomnia, a disorder of initiating and/or maintaining sleep, it is important to apply certain treatment measures. Not only is attention to sleep hygiene important, but such stimulants as caffeine and nicotine must be avoided near bedtime. Regular daily exercise, including stretching and aerobic activity, is a form of treatment that can help to consolidate sleep and to alleviate other symptoms. Biofeedback and relaxation techniques, as discussed in chapter 6, are useful in overcoming problems of initiating sleep.

High levels of arousal associated with racing thoughts, worrying, or rumination may also delay sleep onset. Meditation or guided imagery (see chapter 6) can be used to help the patient relax while focusing thoughts on a neutral or enjoyable target.

Nutritional and Hormonal Therapy for Sleep Disorders

About forty years ago, pharmacological studies suggested that the hormone serotonin may have a role in sleep induction. Later on, experiments in animals showed that destruction of the parts of the brain that housed serotonin-containing nerve cells could produce total insomnia. Partial damage to these areas of the brain caused variable decreases in sleep. The percentage of destruction of these particular nerve cells was correlated with the amount of slow-wave sleep.

It turns out that a nutrient, an amino acid called *trypto-*

phan, is a precursor in the synthesis of serotonin in the brain. Since tryptophan is present in milk—and warm milk seems to help some individuals fall asleep—this amino acid became a popular item at health food stores as the home remedy for insomnia. However, some patients who ingested tryptophan as a dietary supplement developed a syndrome with features of a disease called *scleroderma,* which included skin tightening, pain in joints, muscle aches, and weakness. These patients also developed anxiety, depression, and difficulty learning. Some patients actually died. It was later thought that the deaths were due to a contaminant of tryptophan in the substance they took.

It needs to be pointed out that not everyone who took the drug experienced side effects. By the same token, not everyone experienced relief from insomnia. Tryptophan, needless to say, fell out of favor as a nutritional supplement and treatment for insomnia and was pulled off the shelves. As discussed in chapter 8, foods rich in carbohydrates can also boost serotonin levels in the brain, helping to induce feelings of sleepiness and relaxation.

Tips to Encourage Sleep

Establishing better sleep hygiene is vital in managing the symptoms of fibromyalgia. In our clinic, patients have experienced great success with the following suggestions:

Sleep only as much as needed to feel refreshed and healthy the following day, not more. Curtailing the time in bed seems to solidify sleep; excessively long times in bed seem related to fragmented and shallow sleep.

A regular arousal time in the morning strengthens circadian cycling and leads to regular times of sleep onset.

A steady daily amount of exercise probably deepens sleep; occasional exercise, however, does not necessarily improve sleep the following night.

Occasional loud noises (e.g., aircraft flyovers) disturb sleep even in people who are not awakened and cannot remember them in the morning. Sound-attenuated bedrooms may help those who must sleep close to noise.

Although excessively warm rooms disturb sleep, there is no evidence that an excessively cold room solidifies sleep.

Hunger may disturb sleep; a light carbohydrate snack before bedtime may help you avoid sleep disturbances.

Caffeine in the evening disturbs sleep, even in those who feel it does not.

Alcohol may help tense people fall asleep more easily, but ensuing sleep is then fragmented.

People who awake feeling angry and frustrated because they cannot sleep should not keep trying, but should turn on the light and do something different. You might have a light snack high in carbohydrates, read a book, or watch a television show in another room.

The chronic use of tobacco disturbs sleep.

Another procedure we use to help patients overcome conditioned insomnia is stimulus-control behavior therapy. The goal is to reassociate the bedroom stimuli with sleep rather than with frustration and arousal. To achieve this, patients are told that they are "misusing" their bed if they lie in it awake and frustrated. Richard Bootzin, the behavior therapist who initiated this approach, recommends the following rules:

Go to bed only when sleepy.

Use the bed only for sleeping; do not read, watch television, or eat in bed.

If unable to sleep, get up and move to another room. Stay up until you are really sleepy, then return to bed. If sleep still does not come easily, get out of bed again. The goal is to associate bed with falling asleep quickly.

Set the alarm and get up at the same time each morning, regardless of how much you slept during the night. This helps the body acquire a constant sleep-wake rhythm.

Do not nap during the day.

If the above rules are followed, patients will usually sleep little during the first night. By the second or third night, patients are so tired that they fall asleep on the first or second attempt. Sleep patterns then fluctuate for a few weeks, but gradually the bedroom surroundings again become associated with sleep. However, most patients need a lot of encouragement during this difficult reconditioning period.

Precise diagnosis is essential to establish the existence of fibromyalgia and to distinguish this disease from other sleep disorders. Once the diagnosis is made, a multifaceted approach is then required to ensure restful and healing sleep and may require some combination of supportive psychotherapy, biofeedback-relaxation techniques, physical fitness training, antidepressants, or some other medicine as discussed in chapter 3, along with careful medical supervision by a physician.

8

STEP 6: FOLLOW THE NUTRITIONAL PLAN FOR HEALING

Although there are no specific "magic" foods that are proven to cure fibromyalgia, research has shown that there are some positive nutritional measures you can take to heal your body. Being at the proper weight and eating healthful foods, including those that are low in fat and high in immunity-boosting antioxidants and phytochemicals, work together to help maximize energy and alertness, while possibly minimizing the constant fatigue and lethargy that accompany this syndrome.

Maintaining health and feeling good become increasingly more complicated with chronic diseases like fibromyalgia. Good health is more about the precise balance of a sound body, mind, and spirit than just the absence of disease. There are unique links among the brain, the hormone system, and the immune system. Within this balance, these links make feeling our best a total experience—physical, mental, and emotional. Taking charge of the areas of your health that you *can* control helps to optimize how you feel even in the midst of the aches and fatigue of fibromyalgia.

Taking Control of Your Disease

Eating for wellness is one of the treatment areas that you do have control over. Knowing that you are doing all you can to eat healthily can give you a sense of power to sustain your physical needs and help you cope with the stresses of everyday life and fibromyalgia.

The food choices you make can affect your weight; obesity is a significant public health problem in the United States, as well as in other developed nations. Studies are now being conducted to see if obesity contributes to an impaired immune system. If this is the case, then it is even more necessary that everyone takes control of his or her weight and nutrition.

Nutrients Support Repair of the Body

Nutrients are special compounds found in foods that support the body's repair, growth, and wellness. They include vitamins, minerals, amino acids, essential fatty acids, and water, and the calorie sources of carbohydrate, protein, and fat. Some nutrients can be made by the body (nonessential nutrients) and others must come from the diet (essential nutrients). A deficiency of either type of nutrient may lead to illness if left untreated.

Antioxidants Give Cell Protection

Antioxidants are essential nutrients that help protect your body against life's stressors. Antioxidant food sources are rich in beta-carotene and vitamins C and E. Antioxidants are thought to play a role in the body's cell-protection system and to interfere with aging and the disease process by neutralizing highly reactive and unstable molecules, called free radicals, produced by the body. In research, free radicals have been shown to disrupt and tear apart vital cell structures like cell membranes. Antioxidants have been shown to tie up these free radicals and take away their destructive power, perhaps reducing the risk of a number of chronic diseases and even slowing the aging process. Eating for wellness requires a diet rich in antioxidants.

Some researchers think that antioxidants might help prevent damage in some types of arthritis and boost immune function when a system is under stress. Both are important benefits for patients.

UNDERSTANDING ANTIOXIDANT FOOD SOURCES

BETA-CAROTENE. Beta-carotene, found in apricots, carrots, cantaloupe, pumpkin, and spinach, is converted to vitamin A in the body. Because of a great deal of media attention, most people think of only beta-carotene as having antioxidant properties, but there are many other carotenoid compounds that do also, including:

alpha-carotene (found in carrots, cantaloupe, and
   pumpkin)
gamma-carotene (found in apricots and tomatoes)
beta-cryptoxanthin (found in mangoes, nectarines,
   peaches, and tangerines)
lycopene (found in guava, pink grapefruit, tomatoes, and
   watermelon)
lutein and zeaxanthin (found in beets, corn, and collard and
   mustard greens)

SOURCES OF BETA-CAROTENE

apricots	papayas
broccoli	peaches
cantaloupes	pumpkins
carrots	red peppers
collard greens	spinach
kale	sweet potatoes

tomatoes   winter squash
turnip greens

VITAMIN C.   Vitamin C (ascorbic acid) protects us against infection and aids in wound healing. When the body is under great stress, the blood levels of ascorbic acid have been found to decline. This decline also occurs with age in both men and women.

Vitamin C plays a vital role in boosting levels of the energizing brain chemical *norepinephrine.* Norepinephrine produces a feeling of alertness and increases concentration. A deficiency of vitamin C can therefore influence your mood as well, leaving you less attentive. It is essential to include plenty of vitamin C sources in your diet.

SOURCES OF VITAMIN C

broccoli   oranges
cantaloupes   peppers
grapefruit and   potatoes
   grapefruit juice   strawberries
kiwi   tomatoes

VITAMIN E.   Vitamin E is important to the body for the maintenance of cell membranes, and this vitamin's antioxidant effect may slow age-related changes in the body. There is now evidence that vitamin E plays a role in lowering the risk of coronary heart disease and heart attack. Adults with intestinal disorders of malabsorption may be deficient in vitamin E.

Because this vitamin is taken in through vegetables and seed oils, it is difficult to ingest large amounts, especially if you are following a low-fat diet.

If your diet is low in vitamin E food sources, check with your doctor and see if you should add 200 to 400 IU daily. Supplements can be found at grocery or health food stores and pharmacies.

SOURCES OF VITAMIN E

margarine   vegetable oils
nuts and seeds   wheat germ

Zinc to Resist Infection

Zinc also has antioxidant effects and is vital to the body's resistance to infection and for tissue repair. Many illnesses, such as
some cancers, kidney disease, long-term infection, trauma,
and cirrhosis of the liver, are associated with zinc deficiency.
Medications may also interfere with absorption in the intestines and cause a zinc deficiency.

More research infers that zinc can help to improve the
immune system in elderly people. However, cautions must be
raised as high doses of zinc are toxic and may, in fact, suppress
the immune function. Again, check with your physician for
what is safe in your situation.

Foods high in zinc include seafood, eggs, meats, whole
grains, wheat germ, nuts, and seeds; tea and coffee may hinder absorption.

Choose Plant-Based Phytochemicals

Nutrition research is now revealing that a variety of food
choices can do more than provide optimal nutrient intake. A
varied diet can also provide hundreds of nutrient and non-
nutrient compounds that may be vital to protection from disease. These compounds found in plant-based foods as a group
are referred to as *phytochemicals.*

Phytochemicals appear in all plants. A diet that includes a
variety of grains, fruits, and vegetables should provide these
substances if you vary your choices and methods of food preparation. Although there are phytochemical supplements and
pills, it is better to get your phytochemicals from a varied diet.

TIPS TO BOOST YOUR IMMUNE POWER
- Use a tomato sauce over pasta
- Add tomato sauce to soups and stews
- Add sliced tomatoes to sandwiches and salads
- Add extra vegetables with antioxidants to your dishes
- Throw some greens and carrots in your vegetable soup
- Try a veggie pizza with broccoli and pepper
- Toss some grated zucchini into your next batch of muffins or loaf of bread
- Snack on dried fruits and nuts like apricots and cashews
- Use chopped nuts or wheat germ to top off your yogurt

Because of the wide array of nutrients in foods essential for wellness, including those not yet identified, relying on supplements for good nutrition may limit your intake to just known compounds.

A diet for wellness should contain foods loaded with phytochemicals.

PHYTOCHEMICAL FOOD SOURCES

PHYTOCHEMICAL	FOOD SOURCES	WELLNESS FACTOR
Carotenoids	Carrots, apricots, sweet potatoes	Prevent cancer and heart disease
Indoles	Cruciferous vegetables like cabbage, broccoli, and cauliflower	Prevent breast and uterine cancer
Isoflavones	Legumes, soybeans	Prevent breast and uterine cancer
Lycopene	Tomatoes, red peppers, carrots	Prevent cancer

PHYTOCHEMICAL	FOOD SOURCES	WELLNESS FACTOR
Sulfides (allyls)	Cabbage, onions, broccoli, garlic, brussels sprouts	Prevent cancer

Other Immune Boosters

A great concern to anyone with a chronic illness is avoiding other illnesses. For example, fibromyalgia can make you feel flulike with the muscle aches and fatigue. So getting the flu on top of having fibromyalgia is like a double whammy. What about those who have fibromyalgia and also develop osteoporosis or heart disease? It doesn't have to happen to you, and one way to protect yourself from viruses, infections, and other chronic illnesses is to keep your immune system boosted so it can adequately fight to keep you well.

FLAVONOIDS

Flavonoids (or bioflavonoids) include about four thousand compounds that are responsible for the colors of fruits and flowers. Hosts of experiments on bioflavonoids found in the soft white skin of citrus fruits have suggested that these key nutrients increase immune system activation. These biochemically active substances accompany vitamin C in plants and act as an antioxidant. You can find bioflavonoids in grapefruit, oranges, lemons, and limes. Rose hips, apricots, cherries, grapes, black currants, plums, blackberries, and papayas are other fruit sources of bioflavonoids. Green peppers, broccoli, eggplant, squash, and tomatoes are some good vegetable sources of bioflavonoids. Tea, red wine, and parsley are also good sources.

QUERCETIN

This is a very highly concentrated form of bioflavonoids that is found in citrus fruits, red and yellow onions, and broccoli. Quercetin reduces inflammation associated with allergies and can inhibit the growth of head and neck cancers. Other citrus flavonoids include *hesperidin,* which is said to raise blood levels of the "good" high-density lipoprotein (HDL fats) and lower the "bad" low-density lipoprotein (LDL fats) and triglycerides, and *tangeritin,* which induces apoptosis, or programmed cell death, in leukemia cells, but does not harm normal cells.

GLUTATHIONE

Another nutrient that has been found to strengthen the immune system so it can fight other infections is glutathione. This powerful antioxidant is most plentiful in the red, pulpy area of the watermelon near the rind. It can also be found in cruciferous vegetables.

Five a Day

As you learn to eat for wellness, it is important to follow the nutritional recommendations from the USDA (United States Department of Agriculture), which advises eating five servings

---

ADDING PHYTOCHEMICALS TO YOUR DIET
- Use spinach, shredded cabbage, sliced carrots, and broccoli in your salads
- Add chopped fruits to cereal, yogurt, ice cream, and muffins
- Snack on cut-up carrots, pepper, broccoli, and cauliflower
- Make a quick dip by adding tomato salsa to nonfat yogurt
- Fill your pantry with plenty of herbs and spices like ginger, garlic, chives, and parsley
- Frequently include steamed cabbage, broccoli, or brussels sprouts with meals

---

of fruits and vegetables a day. Through groundbreaking research, this organization has concluded that we are what we eat, and the nutritional components of fruits and vegetables can prevent or even reverse some diseases and conditions. The National Cancer Institute goes one step beyond the USDA's recommendation by encouraging us to eat nine servings of fruits and vegetables (or more) a day for better health.

Whether you opt for five a day or can reach the ultimate goal of nine servings a day, it is important to know why this recommendation is important to maintaining good health. The answer lies in the ability of these food sources to prevent a wide range of chronic diseases and bolster the body's immune power. They provide the basic elements for a healthful diet as high-fiber, low-fat powerhouses of antioxidants and phytochemicals, among many other essential and nonessential nutrients.

EASY WAYS TO ADD FRUITS AND VEGETABLES TO YOUR DAILY DIET

Breakfast: 4 oz. of grapefruit juice (1)
1 bagel with jelly
½ cup skim milk

Snack: 1 cup low-fat yogurt
½ cup raspberries (1)

Lunch: ½ cup spinach salad (1)
tuna sandwich with a sliced
tomato (1)
1 cup skim milk

Dinner: ½ cup broccoli (1)
4 oz. baked chicken breast
½ cup wild rice
rolls
½ cup sherbet

TOTAL FOR DAY: Five servings of fruits and vegetables

To meet the goal for nine fruits and vegetables a day, increase the amount of salad, vegetables, fruits, and juice to reach the total.

Eat Frequently to Boost Energy

Many FMS patients have found that eating frequent mini-meals helps in keeping energy levels higher and also helps to maintain a normal weight. Studies show that eating *more frequently* throughout the day, as opposed to three heavy meals, will boost your metabolism and productivity. Research has found that people who eat two meals or less during the day have a slower metabolic rate (the speed at which your body burns calories, and the rate that we all want to go faster) versus those who eat three or more times a day. Eating frequently will also keep your blood glucose constant so you do not feel irritable or overly hungry.

An easy way to adjust to mini-meals is to break your daily food intake into five or six small meals, spaced every three to four hours throughout the day. Each mini-meal will have about two hundred to three hundred calories. You can adjust these, depending on your total caloric goal.

Your daily menu may look like this:

Mini-meal 1: 1 cup yogurt, 6 oz. juice, 1 slice toast, hot tea

Mini-meal 2: 2 wheat crackers with 1 Tbsp. peanut butter, ½ cup strawberries

Mini-meal 3: 3 oz. water-packed tuna, low-fat mayo, lettuce, tomato, 2 slices bread, 1 apple, tea

Mini-meal 4: ½ banana spread with 1 Tbsp. peanut butter, ½ cup skim milk

Mini-meal 5: 3 oz. baked skinless chicken breast, 1 baked potato with low-fat sour cream, 1 cup steamed broccoli, mineral water

Mini-meal 6: 3 cups air-popped popcorn, ½ cup red grapes

Add Dietary Fiber to Daily Meal Plan

Dietary fiber is one more valuable bonus we get from eating five to nine (or more) servings of fruits and vegetables per day. It is the part of the plant that we can eat but our bodies cannot digest or break down. Fiber moves foods and the toxins they contain quickly through the digestive tract, allowing less time for any possible cancer-causing agents to come in contact with the intestines, colon, or rectum. According to the National Cancer Institute, a diet high in fiber cuts the risk of colon cancer by up to 70 percent and may also lower the risk of kidney stones and gallstones, as well as ease constipation. Fiber ferments in the colon, increasing the amount of oxygen, which in turn diminishes the action of the harmful bacteria. Fresh, whole fruits and vegetables, including the skins, provide the most benefit from fiber. Figs, prunes, and dried beans and peas are also very high in fiber, so include them in the diet on a regular basis.

The National Cancer Institute recommends 25 to 35 grams of fiber per day, yet most Americans eat considerably less than that. About one-fourth of your daily fiber intake should consist of the soluble type fiber found in oats, beans, fruits, and vegetables. The rest of your fiber intake should come from the insoluble type, found in wheat bran and whole grains.

FOODS HIGH IN SOLUBLE FIBER

acorn squash	dates
apples	dried beans
baked potatoes	lentils
blueberries	peas
broccoli	prunes
cabbage	pumpkins
carrots	raspberries
cauliflower	strawberries
citrus fruits	sweet potatoes

You can increase your dietary fiber by adding at least six servings of whole grain breads and cereals, pasta, rice, and dried peas and beans, along with the five to nine servings of fruits and vegetables, to your diet. As you begin to include low-fat, high-complex carbohydrate foods in your diet, you will notice a gradual reduction in your weight. For most patients, this is an appreciated added benefit.

GUIDELINES TO INCREASE FIBER

Eat more legumes that are very high in fiber. Red beans, black beans, great northern beans, and other legumes are high in fiber and have no fat. Don't cook legumes with animal fat.

Eat raw vegetables for snacks. Two carrots will give you a day's supply of vitamin A and provide more than seven grams of fiber.

Read your cereal box at the grocery store. If the cereal has less than three grams of fiber, it probably has little nutrient value.

Add dried fruits to your cereal. Three prunes can give you four grams of fiber.

THE FIBER CONTENT OF SELECTED FOODS (GRAMS)	
1 medium bran muffin	3
1 slice of whole wheat toast	2
1 ounce of raisin bran	4
⅔ cup of oatmeal	4.5
1 medium apple with skin	3
1 medium orange	3
1 medium raw carrot	4
½ cup of cooked kidney beans	7

Keep your vegetables crisp when you cook them. Eat them with skins on to add to the fiber content.

Eat fruits with the skin on for an extra fiber boost.

Top Ten Power Healers

Try to include the following healing foods in your diet each day. Some easy ways include:

Sauté broccoli sprouts with fresh garlic in olive oil.
Add tomato slices to a lunchtime tuna sandwich.
Drink low-fat milk with your meals.
Have a quick snack of soy nuts and hot green tea.
Toss grapes in your spinach salad and serve with a sweet-
and-sour dressing.

BROCCOLI
This green, treelike vegetable is full of indoles, isothiocy-anates, and sulforaphane—phytochemicals that pack a power punch of healing nutrition! If you really want the highest con-centration of these cancer-fighting compounds, get broccoli sprouts at your local health food store. The sprouts have ten to a hundred times more sulforaphane than mature broccoli.

DAIRY PRODUCTS
Low-fat dairy products such as low-fat milk, buttermilk, cheese and cheese products, cottage cheese, ice milk, and yogurt are all important in keeping your body functioning at its peak. The calcium and vitamin D in dairy products help to keep bones strong and prevent osteoporosis and fractures. Studies show that a diet high in low-fat dairy products and fruits and vegetables significantly lowers blood pressure.

FISH

New studies show that eating fish at least once a week can cut the risk of sudden cardiac death. One eleven-year study of 20,551 male physicians found that men who ate fish once a week had half the risk of sudden cardiac death as those who ate fish less than once a month. Although this study focused on men, it wouldn't hurt women to get on the bandwagon! Substances in fish called n-3 fatty acids may have a protective effect against sudden cardiac death, possibly by preventing potentially dangerous arrhythmias or irregular heartbeats. Some heart-healthy fish include anchovies, bluefish, lobster, mackerel, salmon, sardines, scallops, tuna, and whitefish.

GARLIC

Scientific research claims that garlic contains chemicals that act like ACE (angiotensin-converting enzyme) inhibitors, those prescription drugs commonly given to lower blood pressure and protect the heart. Supplements of garlic reduce blood pressure by dilating blood vessels. In fact, some studies have revealed that ingesting as much as one or two cloves of fresh garlic per day can lower mild blood pressure an average of 8 percent in one to three months. Researchers have found that garlic and onions can block formation of nitrosamines. These are powerful carcinogens that target several sites in the body, usually the liver, colon, and breasts.

GREEN TEA

Green tea is a powerful antioxidant and may help in reducing the risk of cardiovascular disease and stroke. Some new studies indicate that it may help in preventing osteoporosis, and other findings reveal that it may help to prevent pancreatic, breast, lung, esophageal, and skin cancers. Researchers report that a nontoxic chemical found in green tea, *epigallocatechin-3 gallate*, acts against *urokinase* (an enzyme crucial for cancer growth). One cup of green tea contains between 100 and 200 milligrams of the antitumor ingredient.

OLIVE OIL

Olive oil is a mono-unsaturated fat that has also been promoted recently as a heart-healthy oil that is preferable to other vegetable oils and margarine. In Mediterranean countries, olive oil is widely used both for cooking and as a salad oil. Breast cancer rates are also 50 percent lower in those countries than in the United States.

RED GRAPES

A new super antioxidant, called activin, has been discovered inside the seeds of red grapes. By-products of the red grape, such as wine, juice, or seeds, may offer significant protection against certain types of cancer, heart disease, rheumatoid arthritis, cataracts, and many other chronic and degenerative diseases. Some studies show that activin is up to seven times more powerful as an antioxidant than vitamins C, E, and beta-carotene. This may explain why red wine is more healthful than white wine in protecting you from heart disease. Recent studies conclude that a glass of wine a day may also reduce the risk of age-associated vision loss.

SOY

Vegetarians have known for years that soy protein is an easy, inexpensive, and healthful alternative to meat. Soy products are dairy-free and do not contain saturated fat. For years, soybeans have played an integral part in Asian culture. In fact, heart disease, breast cancer, prostate cancer, and osteoporosis rates for Asian men and women are much lower than for Americans. In a recent study of one thousand people reported in the *American Journal of Epidemiology* (1996), those who ate soybeans in some form at least once a week had half the risk of developing the polyps that are precursors to colon cancer compared to those who did not eat soybeans.

Isoflavones are phytonutrients found in soy that are converted into phytoestrogens (plant estrogens that are close in structure to the body's form of estrogen) in the body. Although these plant ingredients mimic the hormone estrogen, they appear to have no harmful side effects and can relieve menopausal symptoms that frequently occur because of plummeting estrogen levels. Studies show that soy protein isolate can also effectively prevent the rise in serum cholesterol associated with ovarian hormone deficiency. If you want to increase soy in your diet yet aren't fond of tofu, try such soy-based products as meatless pepperoni, salami, hot dogs, bacon, puddings, and dairy alternatives. Some calcium-rich soy foods include tahini, calcium-set tofu, fortified soy milk, textured vegetable protein, and soy nuts.

SPINACH

Homocysteine has been a big news maker. This naturally occurring blood protein promotes artery clogging, and is a byproduct of meals high in protein. How do you counteract homocysteine? Add more folic acid. Folic acid, which is found in spinach, dramatically lowers elevated levels of homocysteine in the blood. Age-related macular degeneration (AMD), the leading cause of blindness in older people, is also significantly decreased by eating this green vegetable. Spinach is high in folacin, a nutrient crucial during early pregnancy to prevent neural-tube defects in children, and this power vegetable is also rich in beta-carotene, vitamins A and C, and potassium. You can easily get the minimum daily intake of folate (400 mcg) by adding the following to your diet:

Dark green vegetables
Fruits, especially citrus fruits or juices
Whole grains
Enriched breakfast cereals

TOMATOES

Preliminary research confirms that the potent antioxidant lycopene, which is prominent in tomatoes, may be more powerful than beta-carotene, alpha-carotene, and vitamin E. This antioxidant is associated with protection against heart disease and certain cancers such as prostate and lung cancer. Cooking tomatoes releases the lycopene and makes it available for absorption in your body.

Foods for a Calming Effect

As we have discussed above, good nutrition influences our ability to stay healthy and recent research has revealed that what we eat can affect our moods as well. In the past twenty years, hundreds of studies have confirmed a connection between certain foods and our ability to feel calm and alert. Dr. Judith Wurtman, a nutrition researcher at the Massachusetts Institute of Technology, has found that certain foods affect brain chemicals that influence our mood, mental energy, and performance.

These "persuasive" foods are high in carbohydrates, such as breads, cereal, pasta, or sherbet, and raise the level of serotonin in the brain. When serotonin levels rise, we feel calm and upbeat for a period of time. As discussed throughout the book, serotonin is the mood-elevating neurotransmitter; it plays an unknown role in fibromyalgia symptoms, especially with depression and sleep disorders. Studies have shown that by including plenty of foods high in complex carbohydrates in your diet, you can boost the level of serotonin and reap the benefits of feeling calm throughout the day and sleeping more soundly at night.

Even though we have a host of new information on the food-mood connection, finding foods that relieve depressed feelings relies on a personal trial-and-error approach. Using the list of the suggested serotonin-boosting foods below, see which ones make a difference in your symptoms and wellness, and then incorporate these in five to six mini-meals throughout the day to keep blood sugar and energy levels even.

HIGH-CARBOHYDRATE FOODS THAT BOOST SEROTONIN

bagels	pasta
bread	potatoes
cereal	rice
crackers	sherbet
muffins	

Foods to Boost Energy and Alertness

Just as some foods can be used to create a calm feeling during times when you experience great stress or anxiety, other foods can create the opposite effect, making you feel attentive and responsive. Foods rich in protein, like turkey, tuna, or chicken, are also rich in an amino acid called tyrosine. Tyrosine boosts levels of the neurotransmitters dopamine and norepinephrine. Neurotransmitters are the chemicals that send messages from cell to cell. Sophisticated research by Dr. Judith Wurtman at the Massachusetts Institute of Technology has revealed that people are more alert when the brain is producing the neurotransmitters dopamine and norepinephrine. The neurotransmitter serotonin is associated with less anxiety and increased drowsiness. Dopamine and norepinephrine may be produced through the dietary consumption of protein. When we eat protein food, this increases the amino acid tyrosine, which boosts the levels of dopamine and norepinephrine. This, in turn, creates a feeling of alertness and improves our concentration. A protein source should be included in your diet several times a day, especially during those times when you need to clear your mind and boost your energy.

Try the following to see which foods boost stamina and alertness.

HIGH-PROTEIN FOODS RICH IN TYROSINE

legumes and peas   soy products
beef   (soybeans, soy
cheese   granules, soy
fish   milk, etc.)
milk   yogurt
poultry

Repairing the Damage of Fibromyalgia

Protein is also important in building and repairing body tissue and in fighting infection. Too little protein in the diet may lead to symptoms of fatigue, weakness, apathy, and poor immunity. The average-size adult needs 45 to 55 grams of protein a day. More protein is needed if there is fever or infection.

One ounce of meat, chicken, cheese, or fish provides 7 grams of protein; 1 cup of milk provides 8 grams of protein. Therefore 5 to 6 ounces of meat per day and 2 cups of milk provide adequate protein for most adults. Vegetable proteins can make a good substitute for animal protein, if eaten with a complementary starch at the same meal. An example of this would be to substitute 1½ cups of black beans and rice for a 2-ounce portion of meat.

COMPLEMENTARY VEGETABLE PROTEINS

beans and bread   legumes and
beans and rice   grains
corn tortillas and   peanut butter
  beans   and bread

Include Iron-Rich Foods

Some specific nutrient deficiencies can impact on how you feel. For example, if you are not including iron-rich foods in your diet (especially menstruating women), then iron-deficiency anemia can result. Symptoms of fatigue, weakness, shortness of breath, and pallor can compound symptoms of fibromyalgia. Make sure your diet includes plenty of iron-rich foods.

IRON-RICH FOODS
dried apricots
dried beans
enriched or fortified bread and cereals
lean, fat-trimmed cuts of red meat (beef, veal, or lamb)
lentils
prunes
raisins

When eating an iron-rich food from a plant source, include a vitamin C source, such as orange or grapefruit juice, along with it to enhance iron absorption. Vitamin C–fortified apple juice is also a good source.

Minimize PMS with Nutritional and Activity Changes

Because female patients with fibromyalgia tend to suffer with painful menstrual cramps, it is important to minimize premenstrual syndrome (PMS) symptoms through some dietary and activity changes. PMS symptoms may include mild breast tenderness, fluid retention, anxiety, dietary cravings, irritability, and an inability to concentrate. Unfortunately, neither the cause nor the cure for PMS is currently known. However, these measures may help alleviate some of the symptoms.

Eat a balanced diet that includes a variety of complex carbohydrate foods (grains, fruits, and vegetables) and a moderate amount of meat and milk products.

Exercise regularly to reduce stress and keep your body fit. A daily exercise program can decrease PMS symptoms. This lessening of symptoms may be connected with the rise in endorphins that occurs with an intense aerobic workout. Regular aerobic exercise increases one's sense of well-being and decreases fluid retention. It has also been shown to be effective in the treatment of depression.

Avoid alcohol before your menstrual period. Since alcohol is a mood-altering drug, it can compound feelings of depression and hopelessness. Furthermore, many women have a decreased tolerance for alcohol prior to their period, and they may become intoxicated quickly.

Avoid caffeine before and during your menstrual period. Studies have shown that symptoms of PMS increase with the consumption of caffeine-containing beverages. In one study, women who totally abstained from caffeine had a complete resolution of symptoms from PMS.

Reduce excessive sodium and salt in the diet to reduce fluid retention. Excessive sodium can lead to bloating, edema, and fluid weight gain during premenstruation; reducing the sodium in the diet can relieve some of these symptoms. The best approach is to eat more foods naturally low in sodium. This includes fresh fruits and vegetables, cereals, and grains.

Another way is to limit the consumption of high-sodium processed foods and the use of table salt. You can add a splash of lemon juice to a glass of water for a natural diuretic.

If you experience premenstrual symptoms of *hypoglycemia* (low blood sugar), such as fatigue, dizziness, and the shakes, divide your meals into six small mini-meals rich in complex carbohydrates and protein and low in simple sugars.

FOODS HIGH IN SIMPLE SUGARS
cakes
candy and gum
canned fruits in syrup
cookies
frozen yogurt and sherbet
fruit juice
pies
regular sodas and sweetened drinks

FOODS HIGH IN SODIUM
canned meats
canned soups
canned tomato products
canned vegetables
frozen prepared meals (vegetables with sauces, meats, casseroles)
processed meats
salted snacks, such as chips, peanuts, pretzels

Vitamin Supplements

Various vitamins and minerals have also been suggested as effective for treatment of chronic muscle pain. No specific evidence favors any single vitamin or mineral supplement, but if you are in doubt, talk with your physician or licensed nutritionist. Premenopausal women especially need to check for iron deficiency. Even a mild deficiency in iron can make it difficult to get through the day without overwhelming fatigue.

If you do take vitamins to boost your immune power, start with a multiple vitamin without minerals that has the Recommended Dietary Allowance (RDA) as suggested by the American Dietetics Association, and then talk with a nutritionist about your specific vitamin needs.

Omega-3

Some foods have been shown to decrease inflammation in the body, whereas others tend to increase the possibility of inflammation. For example, animal foods contain fats that have been found to increase an inflammatory response. But studies show that eating high-fat fish, such as mackerel, bluefish, or tuna, that contain N-3 or omega-3 fatty acids enables the body to make products that tend to decrease the inflammation.

The most commonly available of these omega-3 fatty acids is found in some fish and fish oil. Although guidelines have not been established regarding supplements of fish oil, EPA (eicosapentaenoic acid) is available in capsules without a prescription. You can ask for these capsules at your drugstore or health food store. Check the instructions on the label as to suggested dosage.

Some patients with arthritis have found improvement in pain and stiffness when they take these capsules for a few months. It is important to use EPA in addition to your basic treatment program, not in replacement of it. When used in the dosage prescribed on the label, no serious side effects are known.

Vegetarians who want to gain this anti-inflammatory benefit can substitute borage seed oil, flaxseed oil, black currant seed oil (BCSO), or evening primrose oil—all said to be helpful in offsetting the inflammation caused by arthritis. These oils all contain gammalinolenic acid (GLA), an omega-6 oil. One study of patients with active rheumatoid arthritis found that BCSO is a potentially effective treatment. Similar studies with fibromyalgia patients have not yet been conclusive.

FISH HIGH IN OMEGA-3

anchovies	salmon
bluefish	sardines
capeline	shad
dogfish	sturgeon
herring	tuna
mackerel	whitefish

An Alkaline Diet

The arthritis diet is an alkaline diet used by some patients for the treatment of osteoarthritis, rheumatoid arthritis, and other conditions where overacidity is thought to play a part. Naturopaths believe that arthritis is caused by the accumulation of toxic acids in the joints. These acids are thought to come naturally from the intestine, and from a failure of the body's metabolism to detoxify them when in excess in the diet. Although dietary changes, such as following a vegetarian diet, have proven to be helpful for patients with rheumatoid arthritis, studies are still inconclusive for those with fibromyalgia.

A Fibromyalgia Diet

Some people with fibromyalgia find that highly acidic foods, such as citrus products, foods in the nightshade family (tomato products, potatoes, eggplant, peppers, tobacco), red meat, cow's milk products, brown and white wheat flour products, sugar-containing foods, coffee, chocolate, and honey, seem to trigger more muscle pain. Eliminating foods to reduce pain is strictly personal and must be done on a case-by-case basis.

If you do try a food-restrictive diet, such as the one offered here, be sure to check with your physician or nutritionist about nutrient supplements that you may need.

AN ALKALINE DIET FOR ARTHRITIS

FOODS TO AVOID	FOODS TO EAT
Red meat	Whitefish, lentils, peas, chicken, eggs (no more than 4 per week)
Cow's milk, cheese, and yogurt	Goat's milk and cheese, soy milk
Brown, white, wheat flour	Oats, brown rice, corn, buckwheat, millet, 100% rye crispbread
Citrus fruit	Tomatoes (no more than twice a week), all other fruit, all vegetables
Dry roasted nuts	All other nuts, especially hazelnut, almond, cashew, and walnut
Sugar and foods containing sugar, syrup, honey	Sugarcane, molasses, dried fruit, sugar-free products
Coffee, decaf coffee, cocoa, tea, alcohol	Grain coffees, herbal teas, unsweetened fruit juices, vegetable juices
Salt, pepper, vinegar	Ruthmol salt, cubes of vegetarian stock
Butter and margarine	Vegetable oil
Chocolate	Carob

In short, good nutrition can help you take an active role in your health and healing. Although there are no guarantees that the foods you eat will heal your fibromyalgia, we do know that good nutrition offers tremendous benefits of increased energy and boosts your immune system to the point where it can cope with the symptoms and fight off other serious illnesses.

9

STEP 7:
SEEK SUPPORT

Living with fibromyalgia is not easy. You may often feel that no one understands the pain, fatigue, and stress that you feel twenty-four hours a day, month after month, year after year. If prolonged, these overwhelming feelings of isolation can become a stumbling block in your quest for wellness, resulting in increased stress, anxiety, and difficulty obtaining restful sleep, not to mention difficulty in keeping healthy relationships.

It does not have to be this way. You can and must seek support to keep fibromyalgia symptoms under control and to feel whole. Whether your main support comes from your physician, a personal friend, a support group of fibromyalgia patients, or even strangers on the Internet, there are caring contacts available—if you seek them.

See an Arthritis Specialist, If Needed

Because fibromyalgia is a rheumatic disease like arthritis, obtaining proper help begins with a specific and accurate diagnosis from a physician who understands the syndrome. I suggest that you start with your primary physician, and then, if needed, seek confirmation from a board-certified rheumatologist, a specialist who diagnoses and treats fibromyalgia daily.

Beyond the initial diagnosis are a host of professionals, from physical therapists and psychologists to sleep disorder specialists and dietitians, who can help you implement the 7-Step Treatment Program as defined in this book.

Consider a Fibromyalgia Support Group

Everyone needs someone to talk to. It may be a good idea to branch out and join a fibromyalgia support group as you experience give-and-take with other sufferers.

Support is necessary for coping with any chronic illness. A support group is geared toward the unique needs of its members and is especially important for fibromyalgia patients. Although support groups are not psychotherapy groups, they do provide patients with a safe and accepting place to vent their frustrations, share their situations, and receive comfort and encouragement from one another. In many such groups, the latest methods of treatment are discussed and members give coping suggestions that you may not be aware of. Assurance is given that someone else knows what you are going through, as people share their struggles in living with this mysterious syndrome. This camaraderie is necessary in order to help you revamp your thought processes. After joining such a group, you may realize that the best experts on a disease are often those who live with it daily, although you should always check with your physician before taking a new remedy.

Fibromyalgia support groups are active around the world. Call the Fibromyalgia Association or the Arthritis Foundation (see Resources, page 215) for more information on support groups in your area. You may also check with your physician or local hospitals to see if such groups are registered. If you cannot find a group, the Fibromyalgia Association or Arthritis Foundation can provide you with information on how to start one yourself.

Try Internet Support Groups

If you would prefer not to join a group, you can find support in the privacy of your home or office on the Internet. You can exchange E-mail with those in foreign countries, who may, in turn, suggest excellent remedies that may not be popular in the United States. When going on-line, check out the World Wide Web for the latest information on fibromyalgia, along with current periodicals and studies on the disease.

On the World Wide Web, you can visit the USA Fibrositis Association home page and the Fibromyalgia news group, among many.

Seek Support from Loved Ones

"I know she is sick, but to be honest, she looks very healthy to me." Tom came to see me about his wife, Claire, to try to find more information on fibromyalgia.

"My boss thinks I'm lazy," Ellen cried during a recent appointment after living with this disease for three years. "I cannot convince him that even though I look normal on the outside, I'm far from being normal on the inside."

Fibromyalgia's reach extends beyond the patient and can affect the entire family. Especially with such a chronic pain-related disease, personal support is necessary, whether from your spouse, family, friends, or coworkers.

It is important to educate your friends and loved ones about your disease, sensitizing them to the symptoms that may come and go but can be immobilizing at times. I have found that not only should the patient be told how to treat this disease, but it is helpful to explain the protocol for treatment to those close to the patient.

Family members can have the best of intentions, but without specific guidance, they sometimes make things worse. Family meetings with a licensed mental health counselor are another way of helping everyone deal with the stress of your disease and may be necessary if lifestyle changes have to be made to accommodate your problems.

Consider a Comprehensive Pain Clinic

If you are still having great pain after months of using the suggested 7-Step Treatment Program in this book, it may be necessary to seek additional support from a comprehensive pain clinic.

Most pain clinics use a multidisciplinary approach to treatment, including medical treatment, physical therapy, and psychological approaches to pain control. As you have learned by reading this book, each of these areas is important and complements the others.

Health care specialists at comprehensive pain clinics usually see more severe cases of deep muscle pain since, by the time of admission, most patients have tried a myriad of other treatments. Even with these more difficult cases, many comprehensive pain clinics across the nation are finding that patients are twice as likely to return to work after comprehensive pain treatment than after other treatments alone. In fact, 40 to 60 percent of the patients with chronic pain treated in comprehensive clinics return to work and report having less pain and improved activity. Considering that these patients had not responded to most other treatments, the figures are encouraging.

HOW TO CHOOSE A PAIN UNIT

The American Chronic Pain Association recommends considering the following guidelines prior to selecting a pain unit. You can contact this organization at P.O. Box 850, Rocklin, CA 95677 or call (916) 632–0922. Your personal physician can refer you to a unit, but many programs accept self-referral.

1. Make sure you locate a legitimate program. Facilities that offer pain management should include several specific components, listed below.

- The Commission on Accreditation of Rehabilitation Facilities (CARF) (telephone: [800] 444–8991) can provide you with a listing of accredited pain programs in your area (your health insurance may require that the unit be CARF-accredited in order for you to receive reimbursement).

- You can also contact the American Pain Society, a group of health care providers, at (708) 966–5595, for additional information about pain units in your area.

2. Choose a good program that is convenient for you and your family.

- Many pain-management programs do not offer outpatient care. Choosing a program close to your home will enable you to commute to the program each day.

3. Learn something about the people who run the program.

- Try to meet several of the staff members to get a sense of the people you will be dealing with while on the unit.
- The program should have a complete medical staff trained in pain-management techniques including:
  - √ Physician (may be a specialist from several different areas but should have expertise in pain management)
  - √ Registered nurse
  - √ Psychiatrist or psychologist
  - √ Physical therapist
  - √ Occupational therapist
  - √ Biofeedback therapist
  - √ Family counselor
  - √ Vocational counselor
  - √ Personnel trained in pain-management intervention

4. Make sure the program includes most of the following features:

Biofeedback training

Counseling

Family counseling

TENS (Transcutaneous Electrical Nerve Stimulation) units

Group therapy

Occupational therapy

Assertiveness training

Regional anesthesia (nerve blocks)

Physical therapy (exercise and body mechanics training, not massage, whirlpool, etc.)

Relaxation training and stress management

Educational program covering medications and other aspects of pain and its management

Aftercare (follow-up support once you have left the unit)

5. Be sure your family can be involved in your care.

- Family members should be required to be involved in your treatment.
- If you choose an out-of-town unit, find out if your family can be involved in your care.
- The program should provide special educational sessions for family members.
- Joint counseling for you and your family should also be available.

6. Also consider these additional factors:

- What services will your insurance company reimburse, and what will you be expected to cover?
- What is the unit's physical setup (is it in a patient care area or in an area by itself)?
- Is the program inpatient or outpatient (when going

through medication detoxification, inpatient care is recommended)?

- Do you understand what will be required of you during
  your stay (length of time you will be on unit, responsibility to take care of personal needs, etc.)?
- Does the unit provide any type of job retraining?
- Make sure that, before accepting you, the unit reviews
  your previous medical records and gives you a complete
  physical evaluation to be sure you can participate in the
  program.
- Obtain copies of your recent medical records to prevent
  duplicate testing.
- Try to talk with both present and past program partici-
  pants to get their feedback about their stay on the unit.

Consider the expense before you go to a pain clinic. It
should be the last resort with fibromyalgia and considered
only if all other methods of treatment fail.

Seeking Support with a Therapist

The fibromyalgia patient deals with pain on a daily basis and
the reason for the pain is genuine—there is something wrong
in the body. For most people, the last thing you want to hear
is, "I think it might be a good idea for you to speak with
someone about the depression and stress you have." You may
conclude that the "someone" is either a psychiatrist, psychologist, or counselor of some type—a "shrink." You may be of-
fended by the implication that the disease is "in your head."
You may even become suspicious that this person does not
believe that you are really feeling the pain and fatigue that you
describe.

It is a fact that all people with pain, whether from fibromyalgia or other diseases, have stress, which in turn makes it
more difficult to handle everyday issues, much less crisis situa-

tions that may arise. One fibromyalgia patient, Sandra, who had severe muscle pain in her shoulders, described her personality as "Dr. Jekyll and Mr. Hyde."

"Depending on whether I've slept well or not, my personality changes with the wind. I warn family and friends not to take offense when I come across irritable or irrational," she said.

Psychological counseling can help you develop appropriate and workable coping strategies to deal with the issues that affect you. It is an accepted treatment for anyone—not just people who have psychological problems or diseases.

If you do seek psychological intervention, not only will you learn new coping methods, but you will also obtain the much-needed support of a professional who understands your feelings and emotions. It is most helpful if your therapist is trained in the area of pain management and/or fibromyalgia.

You may select a one-on-one session with a therapist. These sessions may include specific help with alleviating depression, anxiety, or stress, along with many other problem areas addressed more specifically in the following section. Other sessions may include a meeting with family members or a group session, such as a support group.

Information Organizations and Support Groups

There is also support available from numerous organizations across the nation. These groups can provide you with brochures on fibromyalgia and related problems and assist you with finding a physician, support group, or pain clinic, if needed. See Resources, on pages 213 to 217.

The pressures of living with a chronic disease can overwhelm you, but it does not have to be this way, as support is available. Ask your doctor to recommend professional help and resources, including psychologists, support groups, or other patients who have fibromyalgia and want to help others.

Send away for pamphlets and brochures from national organizations listed in the Resources section of this book, or go online and plug into a support group on the Internet.

Support from others can help you realize that you are not alone in dealing with fibromyalgia and can give new confidence as you learn to handle the daily challenges in a reasonable manner.

10 QUESTIONS PATIENTS ASK ABOUT FIBROMYALGIA

I believe that learning from others who have fibromyalgia is an excellent way to gain control over the disease's long-lasting symptoms. The following commonly asked questions will reinforce your understanding of the disease and the practical and medical responses for coping that you've learned from this book.

Q. I try to eat a varied diet but wonder if I might also need vitamins. Which are recommended?

A. Although your doctor or a certified nutritionist would be the best person to guide you, you may start with the following:

Vitamin C: 250 to 1,000 mg daily
Vitamin E: 200 to 400 IU daily
Multivitamin/mineral: 100 percent of the RDA for most vitamins and minerals
Folic acid: 400 IU daily (usually contained in multivitamin/mineral tablet)
Calcium supplement: 1,000 to 1,500 mg daily
Add other nutritional supplements as suggested by your health care professional.

Q. I was a cross-country runner in college, but in my senior year I was in an automobile accident. Since that time four years ago, I have ached all over from deep muscle pain. My doctor mentioned that I might have fibromyalgia. Do you think it was caused by the accident?

A. The chances are great that it could be related. Researchers in Israel studied people who had undergone severe stress such as military combat situations, severe auto accidents, work accidents, or terrorist incidents. They found that 21 percent of these patients also had fibromyalgia. They concluded that there may be a possible association between stress and pain, such as in fibromyalgia.

Q. I have many symptoms that are similar to those in fibromyalgia, yet my doctor insists that I have chronic fatigue syndrome. How are these ailments different?

A. Chronic fatigue syndrome (CFS) has fatigue that has been present for six months or more, which is often severe enough to cause a patient to go to bed, to not leave the home, or to be unable to work. The symptoms may begin after an illness that seems like a virus or flu, but most patients feel that it started suddenly. Problems sleeping, concentrating, and remembering recent events are common.

Like fibromyalgia, pain and stiffness in the joints and muscles are common. Headaches and fatigue after exercise are also common. Sleep is usually a problem, and many patients find sleep is not restful. Just as with FMS, there are no specific tests available to tell the diagnosis of chronic fatigue syndrome. Your doctor must make the diagnosis based on evaluation of all of your signs and symptoms. The treatment of chronic fatigue syndrome is similar to that of fibromyalgia.

Q. Why does my fibromyalgia seem to act up when the weather gets cold or very humid? My husband says I am imagining this, but I know it's true.

A. The effect of changes in weather is real. Those with arthritis or any type of chronic pain will notice higher levels of aches and pains during inclement weather or when weather fronts pass their locale. In fact, about 60 to 70 percent of patients notice changes in their pain with weather changes.

Fibromyalgia is one of the types of arthritis most sensitive to weather changes. Some researchers even include this as a characteristic part of fibromyalgia. The most common weather changes that can affect pain control are barometric pressure, humidity, and temperature. Most patients find that their pain is worse when these weather conditions change, whether the conditions are good or bad. Some patients feel better with cold and rainy weather with low barometric pressure, whereas others feel worse under the same conditions. Still others may not notice any difference with the weather. Some weather reports now include "pain forecasts" for areas that are more likely to notice changes in arthritis pain and stiffness.

Try the following suggestions when the weather changes and you expect to be affected:

- Treat it like a flare-up of fibromyalgia, and even before it happens, be sure you're doing twice daily moist heat (shower, bath, whirlpool, hot tub).
- Continue to exercise in the shower or immediately after, gradually increasing toward your goal of twenty repetitions of each exercise, twice daily.
- Keep up your walking or bicycling, working up to twenty to thirty minutes each day.
- Continue your medications that have proven to be effective in the past.

- Continue your complementary/alternative treatment program.

Q. How do you know if a new medication or treatment will really work for FMS? I've heard about some miracle cures lately and would love to try one—if I knew they'd work.

A. Although many common health problems like FMS have no cure, there will always be treatments offered by well-meaning family members and friends who want you to have relief of pain and tiredness. Some people will tell you how a new treatment worked for them. These "personal testimonials" might seem appealing. After all, who would want to miss the chance for relief, even if it may not be proven or approved by the FDA?

Nonetheless, the nagging question remains: How can you get the benefit of new treatments for FMS but avoid the bad ones? What if your doctor is needlessly avoiding a good treatment?

You can best protect yourself from wasting both time and money by becoming an expert. Learn about FMS by getting information from your doctor, the library, and the Internet. The information available on the Internet is almost unlimited and can give you a good idea of the current standard and nonstandard or complementary treatments. You can find where to go to get the best available diagnosis and treatment for your FMS. Each source can lead you to other ways to learn more about each treatment. The more you know, the better you will understand FMS, and the better you'll be at helping your doctor decide your own best plan to get the best relief of pain.

A few questions may help you sort out treatments that are more legitimate and safe. Ask:

What are the side effects?
Is it safe for long-term treatment?
Was it tested in trials approved by the FDA?

What has happened to similar treatments over the years?

Even if you aren't sure about a treatment for FMS, if it is harmless and doesn't delay a proper diagnosis and known treatment, it's okay to try it. Many ointments, rubs, and creams are good examples. A copper bracelet for arthritis doesn't hurt and some feel better just by wearing one. But in some areas, remedies such as rattlesnake meat in capsules was found to cause severe illness or death.

Most of our FMS patients have tried one or more types of complementary treatments. Just remember to continue with the treatment methods we know will help, such as moist heat and exercise, while you check out the safe nonstandard treatments. Take advantage of new ideas but avoid those that may cause more harm than good.

Q. I've had fibromyalgia since my early twenties. I'm planning to get pregnant this year and wondered if this will worsen my pain and fatigue.

A. It's good that you are thinking ahead, trying to understand what your body may go through with a change such as pregnancy. In other types of arthritis, such as rheumatoid arthritis, patients often have improvement in pain and stiffness during pregnancy. Unfortunately, most studies have revealed a worsening of the symptoms of fibromyalgia. In fact, most patients feel worse for the first three months after pregnancy, with some studies revealing as many as 80 percent of women having increased symptoms.

Since stress, both physical and emotional, is known to aggravate fibromyalgia, it is not surprising that symptoms can be worse during and after pregnancy. Pregnancy and delivery are high-stress times, both physically and emotionally, with large changes in the levels of estrogen, progesterone, and other hormones. Since the time after a pregnancy can be difficult for mothers even without the added pain of fibromyalgia, it is important to be aware of the possible increase in pain that can occur then, too.

The good news is that there are some steps that can be taken to help reduce stress during and after pregnancy. Make sure you get regular rest periods, two or three times each day for twenty to thirty minutes each time. This will help you improve the quality of the rest of the day and evening. Be sure to use moist heat twice daily (a warm shower or bath, along with gentle stretching exercises). While pregnant, do not use a whirlpool spa or hot water in your bath, as it could endanger the fetus.

Talk with your doctor about the type and use of medications to control pain and stiffness just as you would at other times during the treatment of fibromyalgia. You might try some of the alternative therapies outlined in chapter 6. A gentle massage, the relaxation response, and music therapy are all easy ways to de-stress and can be done during pregnancy. A word of caution: Be sure to check with your doctor before taking any of the herbs listed in chapter 6. And after the pregnancy, if you breast feed, be sure you check with your doctor before you take any medications.

Q. I was diagnosed with fibromyalgia about three years ago. This past week my doctor told me I also have TMJ and must get a dental appliance to wear during sleep. What is TMJ and what can I do to ease the pain in my jaw and ear?

A. TMJ syndrome is very common in women, in fact, from 80 to 95 percent of the cases affect women. It can start as early as the teenage years or in the twenties. Pain is felt in the muscles used for chewing, with areas of localized tenderness, and sensations of popping or clicking. It may be hard to completely open the jaw, due to pain when chewing. Many patients complain of clicking sensations, even though they are also common in otherwise healthy people.

Many experts think clicking sensations alone are not a sign of serious disease.

To relieve the symptoms of TMJ, use moist heat. Slowly exercising the jaw joints and surrounding muscles might help, even though it may seem hard to imagine at first. Exercises can help make your muscles stronger and more flexible, which gives the joints more support.

In some cases, local injections into the trigger points can give relief. These can be done under a local anesthetic in your doctor's office, and the injections are sometimes combined with a cortisone derivative. Relief may last hours to days and may increase with a second or third injection.

As your doctor suggested, bite adjustment with an oral appliance may give some relief, but you may want to get a second opinion. Many experts find that bite adjustments do not give lasting relief associated with TMJ pain.

Medications such as Elavil (amitriptyline) and Tofranil (imipramine) are used in treatment of this type of pain, and muscle relaxants such as Flexeril may give relief. Although some patients do resort to surgery on their TMJ, most experts would consider this a last resort for difficult cases only.

Talk to your doctor again. Sometimes, psychological evaluation for stress management may be helpful.

Q. Is it normal for my symptoms to flare up the week before my menstrual period? I am achy, exhausted, and toss and turn at night for about five days before my period. What can I do to relieve this?

A. It is very common to have aggravation of symptoms during the week before your menstrual period starts. Knowing that this is true, you can take "preventive" measures to avoid worsening of the symptoms.

Stay with your twice-daily moist heat, exercise, and stretch each day, and continue with the medications your doctor has prescribed. Read pages 167 to 169 in chapter 8 and follow the suggestions for dietary control to ease PMS symptoms. Perhaps more importantly, watch your schedule. Try to avoid a high-stress week with too many commitments. Staying home during the evenings and relaxing the week prior to your period may help you to unwind and sleep more soundly. Try one of the calming herbs such as chamomile (chapter 6) in a warm tea before bedtime, and see if this may give relief.

Q. I have lived with fibromyalgia symptoms for six years, and my doctor recently diagnosed it as a specific disease. She sent me to a fibromyalgia support group in our city, and thirty-two of the thirty-eight members were women around my age (age forty-nine). Does this mean that fibromyalgia is a middle-aged woman's disease?

A. It is really common to be bothered by the feelings of fibromyalgia for years before an exact diagnosis is made. Once the diagnosis is made, however, the picture becomes clear. Only then can proper treatment begin.

Support groups for fibromyalgia are a great source of information. This is a good way to keep up with the latest research and treatments available. Dealing with fibromyalgia alone can be discouraging; it helps to talk openly with others who have dealt with the problem successfully. Also, you may be able to help others.

Yes, it is a fact that most fibromyalgia patients are women, but it can happen in men. About 90 percent of patients (nine in ten) are women, commonly in the middle years of life.

Q. I keep hearing that this is a woman's disease, yet I am a six foot two male who was recently diagnosed with fibromyalgia. Could there be a hormonal problem that is causing this to happen to my body? If so, what treatment would be effective?

A. Although it is true that the vast majority of cases of fibromyalgia happen in women, it is also true that men suffer from this disease as well. The specific causes are not known. In our clinic, we do see fibromyalgia in men at times and some of them have had a severe injury to the back, such as a ruptured disc in the lumbar spine, months or even years before.

There is no evidence that hormones play a role in fibromyalgia in men. The treatment is the same for both men and women, and by staying on my 7-Step Treatment Program, you should obtain relief.

Q. I was diagnosed with fibromyalgia after having great pain stemming from a hysterectomy. I had pain when I awoke, and then more pain throughout the day. Then it seemed as if my bladder completely shut down. I was rushed to the emergency room for a catheterization and was told it was part of fibromyalgia. Have you ever heard of this happening?

A. Fibromyalgia can begin after a very stressful situation, an injury, or a serious illness. Some women have found that it began after a hysterectomy. Remember, the causes are just not known. Many problems other than pain and stiffness can result, such as abdominal pain, bloating, constipation and diarrhea, and irritable bowel syndrome (IBS).

Also, as discussed on page 26, urinary frequency, the urge to urinate, and pain on urination can come with fibromyalgia. There is no special treatment other than the treatment of the disease itself and certain medicines that can help the bladder control.

Talk to your doctor to be sure you have the best combination of medicines to control the symptoms of this disease.

Q. My family practitioner is treating me for fibromyalgia, but I feel that I need a specialist. What type of doctor would you recommend for this disease? Are there certain tests I will need?

A. See your family doctor first, but if your fibromyalgia is not improved after a reasonable amount of time (say a few months), then yes, it is a good idea to ask for an opinion from a rheumatologist. Rheumatologists deal with arthritis and related diseases. They treat many patients with fibromyalgia. This specialist will review your diagnosis and coordinate the plan for treatment.

The diagnosis of fibromyalgia is still made from an examination and talking with the patient. A few blood tests and X rays will help to eliminate other types of arthritis. This is important to be sure that no other specific treatments will be needed. If the rheumatologist agrees with the diagnosis of fibromyalgia, a plan for treatment can be made.

Q. After a lengthy bout with the flu, my seventeen-year-old daughter was diagnosed with fibromyalgia. Is this common?

A. Fibromyalgia does happen in teenagers. Although uncommon, it causes the same pain, stiffness, and fatigue that adults experience. It usually improves slowly over time. The course of treatment may be helped by a regular program of moist heat, exercises, and medication, as discussed in chapter 3. Just as in adults, fibromyalgia in teenagers seems to follow a severe injury or illness, but the exact reason why is not known.

Q. Does taking estrogen have anything to do with fibromyalgia? After a complete hysterectomy at age thirty-five, my doctor put me on estrogen replacement. Within one year, I developed horrible muscle pain and fatigue that would not end, even with bed rest. Was it the estrogen? If so, what should I do?

A. There is no good evidence that the hysterectomy or the estrogen treatment is the cause of fibromyalgia, although fibromyalgia does occur in some women after a hysterectomy. The surgery as well as the estrogen treatment are common events in many women. Unless your doctor advises otherwise, you can continue your estrogen treatment without fear of aggravating your fibromyalgia.

However, in some patients with fibromyalgia, there does seem to be a major illness, injury, or emotional stress just before the start of their symptoms. It is not known how these events seem to trigger fibromyalgia. Perhaps future research will bring this answer to light.

Q. Fibromyalgia has taken over my life and is taking over my family's life as well. Is there a cure for this, or will it continue to cause pain forever? Growing older with all this pain does not seem appealing. What does research show for the future?

A. The chronic pain and fatigue can certainly take over your life. It can cause avoidance of your usual activities, less exercise, more pain, and a vicious cycle of further withdrawal, which can lead to depression. The chronic pain of fibromyalgia can change your personality, making it difficult to get along with those you love.

Although there is no cure and no prediction about how long the disease will take to run its course, it's important that your family shares in your disease. When you are tired, stressed, and in pain, it affects how your family feels and acts.

A big problem in fibromyalgia is that the patient does not appear to be sick. There are few outward signs of pain. The frustration from your inability to keep up with your activities shows to others in the way you act. It is a good idea to see a clinical psychologist or psychiatrist for tips on stress management. This professional can be invaluable in helping you deal with the stress of chronic pain.

Right now, there is no cure for fibromyalgia in sight, but

good treatment is available and will work, if you stick to the 7-Step Program. Most patients eventually improve with treatment. Your goals might be to have a reasonable relief of the pain and tiredness so that you can get around and do the things you need to do each day.

Q. I am the mother of three daughters and was recently diagnosed with fibromyalgia. Does this mean that my daughters will also be subject to this disease? Are there prevention methods?

A. If you have the diagnosis of fibromyalgia, it does not mean that your daughters are also destined to be sufferers. The causes of fibromyalgia are unknown. Since there are no known ways to prevent fibromyalgia, I suggest that you simply keep up a good exercise program, including maintaining your cardiovascular fitness, and encourage your daughters to do the same. There is some evidence that an ongoing exercise program, including good conditioning, may make a person more resistant to fibromyalgia.

Q. I started the daily exercise program, but on some days just getting out of bed is a chore. Then, after I exercise, I ache even more. Should I push myself even when the pain and fatigue are unbearable?

A. Most patients with fibromyalgia feel stiff on awakening in the morning. It may even take an hour or more to loosen up. These feelings are very much a part of the disease. Usually, when there is relief of other symptoms with treatment, there is also improvement in the morning stiffness.

It is also typical to have worsening of the aching and pain after exercise. This is a big problem, since it can make patients avoid exercise, an important healing component of the 7-Step Treatment Program. In our clinic, we suggest that patients do their best to keep up the regular exercise program, on good and bad days.

Aerobic exercise, such as an exercise class, walking, bicycling, or swimming, should be continued daily, if possible. On bad days, you might do a little less, but try not to stop completely. Gradually increase back to your old level as soon as you feel less pain.

Remember, on days when you feel better, you may be tempted to totally skip exercise. Don't let this happen! Regular exercise can help you have more good days in the future.

Q. I started NSAIDs for the muscle aches of fibromyalgia, but they did little for the pain. Without purchasing a host of medications, is there a way to tell which medication will help most?

A. NSAIDs (nonsteroidal anti-inflammatory drugs) may not help at all in fibromyalgia. This is because there is little inflammation present in the tissues, if fibromyalgia is the only problem. But these medications may also be used as pain relievers, so you may try them for that reason.

There are more than twenty NSAIDs available on the market. Most people find one that works without side effects, but it may be necessary to try a number of different types to find the one that is best. Ask your doctor to make a suggestion. In our clinic we try to provide our patients with manufacturer samples. When a patient finds a sample medication that works effectively, then the medication can be purchased.

If you notice any new problems, such as nausea, then check with your doctor to see if you should continue using this NSAID.

Q. My doctor told me that my constant pain and fatigue were caused by fibromyalgia, even though my lab tests were normal. How can she be sure that this is fibromyalgia and not some other disease?

A. There are no specific blood tests or other tests that can definitely make the diagnosis of fibromyalgia, but these tests can help rule out certain diseases. The diagnosis is made by the symptoms you express to your doctor: the widespread pain, the trigger points, typical fatigue, depression, and other problems, as discussed in chapter 2. Some of the most common problems that may also be present with fibromyalgia include osteoarthritis, rheumatoid arthritis, and other types of arthritis or thyroid disease. Each of these problems has specific symptoms and tests for diagnosis.

Q. Can't I speed up the course of fibromyalgia? I've had this disease for seven years and see no end in sight.

A. Fibromyalgia can last for years, but there are definite steps you can take to control the symptoms. There is no cure at this time, but the program of moist heat, exercises, medication, and other measures can make the pain tolerable. If you can control your pain and do most of your usual activities, you can win against fibromyalgia.

Many researchers have found that after a few years, the limitations from fibromyalgia are fewer. Many people still have some pain but not the severe and widespread pain and fatigue that was present in earlier years. One study found 24 percent of patients developed excellent control of their symptoms. About 50 percent of patients in the same study experienced more frequent pain-free periods. You can speed up the improvement of the disease with the 7-Step Treatment Program described in this book.

Q. What about moist heat in the treatment of fibromyalgia? I bought a Jacuzzi in hopes that this would help alleviate my constant pain.

A. I don't know of anyone who has not felt totally relaxed after spending time in a Jacuzzi or whirlpool bath. Hot baths are part of one of the oldest methods of alternative treatments for chronic pain associated with arthritis, specifically fibromyalgia. The Romans built baths to provide warm pools for treatment, and the theory behind these baths is just as useful today. The moist heat gives soothing relief to painful muscle aches and provides comfort just as in today's treatments. Many times after relaxing in a whirlpool or Jacuzzi, you are able to do your exercises easily, without as much muscle pain.

Q. Why do you keep saying to exercise when I can hardly get out of the chair? I cannot imagine starting a walking or biking program with the pain I have.

A. Many researchers find exercise to be one of the most important parts of the treatment of fibromyalgia, because it can help improve endurance and strength. Most fibromyalgia patients have not exercised regularly for some time because of the pain and are out of condition. However, in treating hundreds of patients with fibromyalgia, we have learned that those who start and continue an exercise program are much more likely to see their symptoms improve.

Usually, the most difficult part is starting the exercise program when you are stiff and in pain. Two types of exercise are helpful. One is endurance exercise, which gives good cardiovascular exercise and improves fitness. This can improve your ability to accomplish daily activities, reduce stress and anxiety, and help with depression.

How do you start endurance exercise? Simply make yourself start walking every day. Walk a short distance, one that you can easily accomplish, and gradually increase that distance. Or use an electronic treadmill indoors and slowly increase the time you spend on the machine.

The second type of exercise used to treat fibromyalgia is muscle-strengthening exercise. These simple exercises, described in chapter 4, can be done at home. Muscle-strengthening exercise achieves two goals: Stronger and more flexible muscles are less likely to become painful and stiff with daily activity; and stronger muscles are less likely to become tired and fatigued with activity.

Q. A friend of mine who also has fibromyalgia mentioned trying DMSO for pain relief. What is DMSO and how is it used? Is it safe?

A. DMSO (dimethyl sulfoxide) is sold in an impure form in some hardware stores and has been used to treat illnesses in horses for years. In humans, DMSO has been used by athletes to treat injuries to muscles and tendons. It is a liquid that is absorbed into the system when applied to the skin. Side effects include strong, garlicky breath odor and occasional skin irritation where it was applied. If DMSO is injected into a vein, it is very dangerous and can cause liver and other internal organ damage. This should never be done.

Although the U.S. Food and Drug Administration (FDA) has not approved DMSO for use in treating arthritis or bursitis, it has found that DMSO might be helpful in relieving pain caused by bursitis, acute injuries, and possibly rheumatoid arthritis. DMSO is used by some fibromyalgia patients. In my clinic, I see little use among fibromyalgia patients, but I do not object if it is used carefully and gives relief.

Q. What about usage of over-the-counter creams, liniments, and lotions for muscle pain relief with fibromyalgia? Are these harmful?

A. Creams, liniments, and lotions are widely advertised and used for the pain of arthritis and other conditions. Many types are available at your drugstore and at health food stores. They are not harmful when used properly and can be continued if you feel improvement in muscle pain.

One newer topical cream, capsaicin, sold over the counter under various brand names, such as Capsaicin or Zostrix, has been found to be quite beneficial in the few existing studies. One particular capsaicin lotion is available in a roll-on applicator and is sold as Capsin (ask your pharmacist for information on this product).

Capsaicin has an active ingredient derived from red chili peppers. When nerve endings in the body are touched by capsaicin, they produce *substance P,* a neurotransmitter that carries pain messages to the brain. Repeated applications of capsaicin results in fewer pain messages to the brain. Although this cream can cause warmth or a burning sensation, it does not cause blistering, and the burning feeling usually decreases the longer the cream is used.

Q. My friend told me about a cream that is only found at health food stores that is made from an herb. Do you know anything about this?

A. Boswellian Cream can be found at some health food stores and has been used for centuries to treat pain-related ailments. This cream is made of four triterpene acids from the herb *Boswellia serrata,* which has been found to bring temporary relief to minor aches and pains associated with arthritis.

Use this cream with caution, as it does produce mild inflammation and redness to the skin when applied, supposedly in order to achieve its healing properties. A loose bandage should be applied after the cream. Boswellian Cream is for external use only; if your skin becomes inflamed, stop its usage.

Q. I'm trying to use complementary treatments in controlling stress. More specifically, I've started a regular program of guided imagery, along with progressive relaxation and deep breathing. How will I know if this is working?

A. Each person reacts differently, and some forms of mind/body therapy will be successful in some patients and less useful in others. The best results happen when the most effective methods for each patient are used for symptom relief. As always, everyone is different. The important factor is to choose those that work for you and launch out in a regular, daily program of relaxation. Monitor your heart rate as you do this. Does the relaxation help you feel calm and at ease? Continue to practice the technique(s) that you choose until you are able to elicit the relaxation response anytime during the day, especially during stressful moments.

Q. You keep emphasizing the importance of a "combination" treatment program. What exactly does this mean?

A. Let me answer that by using two interesting case studies. Patty epitomized the typical fibromyalgia patient. This thirty-seven-year-old mother maintained a very successful home-based business while caring for her four children. She volunteered at her church and helped teach computer at her children's school two afternoons a week. Although she never found time to exercise, Patty was able to maintain a normal weight simply from the nervous energy she burned balancing so many responsibilities . . . until she was diagnosed with fibromyalgia.

"It started with unending fatigue after getting the flu last winter," she said. "I kept thinking that if only I could get more sleep I would feel well, but the tiredness wouldn't go away. Then I began to feel achy all over, day after day. Sometimes I got a grinding sound in my neck when I moved it. My neck began to feel stiff all the time, as well as both shoulders, and when I touched my neck, it felt warm. My muscles would be so sore that it felt like I had exercised for hours the day before, but I hadn't. Even my scalp hurt."

Patty didn't have time to tolerate the interruption of fibromyalgia's symptoms in her busy life. I recommended her to a stress clinic in town, where she worked with the therapists using biofeedback, guided imagery, and the relaxation response. Her physical therapist referred her to a licensed massage therapist, and she went for weekly muscle massages. After three months of treatment, medication that helped her to achieve restful sleep, and a regular exercise program, Patty was feeling hopeful that she could live a normal life in spite of her disease.

Patty's experience illustrates what I have found to be true, that a combination treatment program can assist a patient in decreasing stress and pacing her lifestyle so that the symptoms of fibromyalgia are diminished or managed.

When forty-six-year-old Marilyn came to see me for an evaluation, she had experienced fibromyalgia symptoms for three years. "The symptoms began around the time my last son left for college," she told me. "At that time, I was very anxious and mildly depressed. My husband, Ray, was fully involved in his career and both boys were away at school. All I had to occupy my time was cleaning the house each day and waiting for Ray to come home from work."

Marilyn told of feeling stiffness and pain in her arms and hands, especially her right hand and thumb. She also had a pinching pain in her left hip, making it difficult to lift her foot to walk. Fibromyalgia also caused painful cramps and sharp, stabbing pains in her left calf. Her toes on the same side would suddenly pull under and cramp.

After an evaluation, I realized that Marilyn had many influences at work in her. Not only was she dealing with the symptoms of fibromyalgia, she was also confronted with what many call the "empty nest syndrome." But this woman did not seek pity. Instead, she sought the assistance of an excellent psychologist, who helped her learn some of the relaxation techniques described in chapter 6. She found music therapy and deep abdominal breathing especially helpful, particularly during stressful times.

Using a combination of treatment, including medication, exercise, moist heat, and the mind/body approach to healing, Marilyn was able to find relief. Choosing any one component of the treatment program alone will not give such outstanding relief. That is why I constantly encourage a total combination treatment program.

APPENDIX: SUGGESTED EXERCISES FOR FIBROMYALGIA PATIENTS

The following exercises are designed to build flexibility and strength in the neck, shoulders, and back. It is important to work toward a goal of doing these exercises twice a day, twenty repetitions each. At first you may only be able to do one to two repetitions of each exercise. That's a reasonable start. But as you gain strength and mobility, move into a twice-daily, twenty-repetitions-each routine. If you have any pain or unusual feeling, stop the exercise and contact your physician.

Sometimes it is helpful to have some gentle assistance from a family member or friend. Your physician or physical therapist can show you how.

A word of caution: Do not hold your breath while performing any exercise. If you feel pain with any of the suggested exercises, stop the exercise and discuss it with your physician.

Neck Range-of-Motion Exercises

It is important to build strength in the neck as well as improve its mobility and flexibility. Because fibromyalgia causes stiffness and pain, these range-of-motion exercises will enable your body to perform more effectively. Although flexion should be done while standing, the rest of the neck exercises can be performed sitting or standing, whichever is more comfortable for you.

FLEXION

While standing, look down and bend your chin forward to your chest. If you feel stiffness or pain, do not force the movement. Go as far as you can without straining yourself. If your muscle pain worsens with this or any exercise, stop until you have talked to your physician or physical therapist.

EXTENSION

Look up and bend your head back as far as possible without forcing any movement.

LATERAL FLEXION

Tilt your left ear to your left shoulder (but do not raise the shoulder). If you feel pain or resistance, do not force the motion.

Now tilt your right ear to your right shoulder, just as you did for the left ear (see figure A.1).

Figure A.1. Lateral flexion.

ROTATION

Turn to look over your left shoulder. Try to make your chin even with your shoulder. Go as far as is comfortable, but do not force the movement.

Now turn and look over your right shoulder, as with the left.

Neck Isometric Exercises

Neck isometric exercises are more advanced exercises to help strengthen the muscles of the neck, which is most important in fibromyalgia. Try these gently and gradually after range of motion of your neck is improved as much as possible. Again, do not hold your breath.

ISOMETRIC FLEXION

1. Place hand on forehead. Try to look down while resisting the motion with your hand. Hold for six seconds, counting out loud.
2. Place your hands on the back of your head. Try to look up and back while resisting the motion with your hands. Hold for six seconds, counting out loud.

ISOMETRIC LATERAL FLEXION

Start with your head straight. Place your left hand just above your left ear (see figure A.2 on page 205). Try to tilt your head to the left but resist the motion with your left hand. Hold for six seconds, counting out loud.

Now place your right hand just above your right ear. Try to tilt your head to the right but resist the movement with your right hand. Hold for six seconds, counting out loud.

Figure A.2. Isometric lateral flexion.

ISOMETRIC ROTATION

Place your left hand above your ear and near your left fore-head. Now try to look over your left shoulder, but resist the motion with your left hand. The hand should not be placed on the jaw. Hold for six seconds, counting out loud.

Now place your right hand above your ear and near your right forehead. Try to look over your right shoulder, but resist the motion with your right hand. Hold for six seconds, count-ing out loud.

Shoulder Range-of-Motion Exercises

The following five range-of-motion exercises will increase the flexibility of the shoulders and arms. Increasing the number of exercises will increase the strength of the arms.

SHOULDER EXTERNAL ROTATION

This exercise increases the motion you use to comb your hair. You may sit, stand, or lie down to do these exercises.

Clasp your hands behind your head. Pull your elbows together until they are as close as possible in front of your chin. Separate the elbows to the side as much as possible.

Repeat this, gradually increasing to five, then ten, then up to twenty repetitions. You may repeat these two or three times daily.

SHOULDER INTERNAL ROTATION

Shoulder internal rotation increases the flexibility of the shoulders. Using the same motions women use to fasten a bra in the back or men use to put a wallet in a back pocket, move your arms behind your back, as shown in figure A.3 (see page 207). This exercise is best done standing and is often done in the shower using a washcloth to wash your upper back and a towel to dry it.

Put your hand behind your back, and then put the other hand behind your back and cross the wrist as shown in the picture. Return the hands to rest at your side.

Repeat this twice daily, gradually increasing to five, then ten, then up to twenty repetitions per session.

SHOULDER FLEXION

Shoulder flexion holds both arms down at your sides. Raise the left arm straight up and reach overhead toward the ceiling. Now do the same with the right arm. Continue this motion as you alternate left-right-left-right.

Repeat twice daily, gradually increasing to five, then ten, then up to twenty repetitions per session.

SHOULDER ABDUCTION

Raise both arms straight out away from your sides, and then raise each arm overhead toward the ceiling and up above your

Figure A.3. Shoulder internal rotation.

head. It doesn't matter whether you do this palm-up or palm-down.

If it's painful to do this exercise while sitting or standing, you can also do it lying on your bed, using a stick (a broom handle will do). As you raise your arms, hold the stick with both hands and keep your arms straight, up over your head as far as possible. The strength of the less painful arm will help the painful arm move more easily.

Repeat this exercise, gradually increasing to five, then ten, then twenty repetitions, two or three times a day.

Once you have mastered the exercise, go to part two of this exercise, which involves raising your arms out to your side, one at a time, then making big circles slowly.

Repeat this exercise, gradually increasing to five, then ten, then twenty repetitions, two or three times a day.

SHOULDER GIRDLE ROTATION

This exercise can be done in a sitting or standing position and is fun to do during the day to relieve neck and shoulder tension and maintain shoulder girdle flexibility.

Roll shoulders in a forward circle, and raise shoulders toward the ears in a shrugging motion. Then, roll shoulders back and your chest out, as in a military stance. Lower the shoulders and bring them forward. Think of it as a simple shoulder roll in a circle. Now reverse the process, rolling your shoulder girdle in a backward circle.

Repeat this exercise, gradually increasing to five, then ten, then twenty repetitions two or three times a day, if possible.

Back Exercises

As you do the following strengthening exercises, it is very important that you breathe properly while holding a position. Counting to six out loud will enable you to do this easily. If you experience shortness of breath, stop and talk to your doctor or physical therapist.

CHEEK TO CHEEK

This is a convenient exercise because you can do it anywhere, anytime, and practically in any position. It strengthens the muscles of the buttocks that help support the back and the legs. When sitting, you will actually rise up out of the chair because of the contraction of the muscle groups in the buttocks.

Press your buttocks together and hold for a six-second count. Relax and repeat. Gradually increase up to five, then ten, then twenty repetitions.

PELVIC TILT

This is one of the best exercises you can do to strengthen your abdominal muscles, which in turn help support your back. It will also help tone your stomach muscles. Do this exercise lying on your back in bed or on the floor, whichever is more comfortable.

Relax and raise your arms above your head. Keep your knees bent. Now comes the tricky part! Tighten the muscles of your lower abdomen and your buttocks at the same time to flatten your back against the floor or bed. Hold the flat back position for a six-second count. Now relax and repeat.

Repeat this exercise two or three times to start and work gradually to five, then ten, then twenty repetitions twice a day.

If you have trouble, contact your physical therapist or physician and have him or her demonstrate the exercise.

BRIDGING

This exercise strengthens the muscles in the back.

Lie on your back on the floor or in bed and bend your knees. Now lift your hips and buttocks off the bed or floor four to six inches, forcing the small of the back out flat; and tighten the buttock and hip muscles to maintain this position (see figure A.4 below). Hold this position for a count of six seconds. Relax and lower your hips and buttocks to the floor or bed.

Figure A.4. A bridging exercise.

Repeat this exercise, gradually increasing up to five, then ten, then twenty repetitions as tolerated. Repeat twice daily, if possible.

PARTIAL SIT-UP

This is one of the more vigorous exercises. Its purpose is to build abdominal strength, which will give the back greater support. To do this exercise, lie on your bed or on the floor, whichever is more comfortable. Lie on your back with your knees bent. Raise your head and shoulder blades off the floor or bed (see figure A.5 below). Hold that position for a six-second count. Slowly return to the beginning position. Repeat.

Start this exercise slowly, with one or two repetitions, until your body adjusts. Gradually increase to five, then ten repetitions.

BACK EXTENSION

For this exercise to strengthen the back muscles, lie on your bed or on the floor in a prone (stomach-down) position. A pillow may be used under the stomach to help make this position more comfortable.

Raise your head, arms, and legs off the floor. Do not bend your knees. This must be done with your body straight in extension. Hold for six seconds while you count out loud. Relax and repeat.

Figure A.5. A partial sit-up exercise.

Gradually increase up to five, then ten repetitions. If you experience discomfort, check with your physician or physical therapist before you continue.

CAT-CAMEL

Do not do this exercise for strengthening the back muscles if you have very painful knees, ankles, or hands, as it places pressure on these areas.

The position for this exercise is a crawling position (see figure A.6 below). Hands must be directly under your shoulders. Take a deep breath and arch your back as a frightened cat does, lowering your head. Hold that position for six seconds, counting out loud. Now exhale and drop the arched back slowly, raising your head.

Start this exercise slowly with one or two repetitions. Increase up to five and then ten repetitions, if possible.

WALL PUSH

This exercise is good for the back because it encourages the body extension positions.

Stand spread-eagle, with your hands against a wall. Now arch your back inward slowly.

Gradually increase repetitions from one to five or more.

Figure A.6. A cat-camel exercise.

This exercise is fun because you can do it anytime you feel you need a good body stretch. Repeat two times daily.

BACK FLEXIBILITY

Lie on your back on the floor with knees bent and feet flat on the floor. Raise hands toward the ceiling. Now move arms and head to the right, while the knees move to the left. Reverse the above, then repeat. Gradually increase up to five and then ten repetitions twice daily.

BICYCLING

Lying on your back, move your feet and legs in the air as if you were riding a bicycle. Count to six and relax. Repeat, then gradually increase to five and then ten repetitions once or twice daily, if tolerated.

RESOURCES

Aids for Arthritis
3 Little Knoll Court
Medford, NY 08055
(609) 654–6918

Alternative Medicine Political
Action Committee, Inc.
1718 M St., #205
Washington, DC 20036

American Academy of
Environmental Physicians
Box CN 1001–2001
New Hope, PA 18938
(913) 642–6062

American Academy of Medical
Acupuncture
5820 Wilshire Blvd., Suite 500
Los Angeles, CA 90036
213–937–5514
(800) 521–AAMA
Web site:
www.medicalacupuncture.org

American Academy of Pain
Management
13947 Mono Way, #A
Sonora, CA 95370
(209) 533–9744

American Alliance of Aromatherapy
P.O. Box 309
Depoe Bay, OR 97341
(800) 809–9850

American Association of Alternative
Medicine, Inc.
1000 Rutherford Road
Landrum, SC 29356

American Association of
Naturopathic Physicians
601 Valley Street, Suite 105
Seattle, WA 98109
(206) 298–0126
Fax: (206) 209–0129

American Association of Oriental
Medicine
433 Front Street
Catasauqua, PA 18032
(610) 266–1433

American Chiropractic Association
(ACA)
1701 Claredon Blvd.
Arlington, VA 22209
(703) 276–8800
(800) 986–4636
Web site: www.amerchiro.org

American Chronic Pain Association
P.O. Box 850
Rocklin, CA 95677
(916) 632–0922

American College of Rheumatology
60 Executive Park S., Suite 150
Atlanta, GA 30329
(404) 633-3777

American Dietetic Association
(800) 366–1655

American Holistic Medical
Association
6728 Old McLean Village Drive
McLean, VA 22101
(703) 556-9728

American Massage Therapy
Association
820 Davis Street, Suite 100
Evanston, IL 60201
(847) 864–0123
Web site: www.amtamassage.org

American Osteopathic Association
142 East Ontario Street
Chicago, IL 60611
(800) 621–1773

American Physical Therapy
Association
1101 17th Street NW, Suite 1000
Washington, DC 20036
(202) 457–1115

American Preventive Medical
Association
459 Walker Road
Great Falls, VA 22066
(703) 759–0662

American Psychiatric Association
(202) 682–6000

American Psychological Association
(202) 336–5700

American Self-Help Clearinghouse
St. Clares–Riverside Medical
Center
25 Pocono Road
Denville, NJ 07834
(201) 625–7101

American Sleep Disorders
Association
1610 14th Street, Northwest
Suite 300
Rochester, MN 55901

Anxiety Disorders Association of
America
6000 Executive Blvd., Suite 513
Rockville, MD 20852
(301) 231–9350

Arthritis Foundation
1314 Spring Street
Atlanta, GA 30309
(800) 283–7800
(404) 872–7100

Arthritis Society
250 Floor Street East, Suite 901
Toronto, Ontario
Canada M4W 3P2
(416) 967–1414

Association of Applied
   Psychophysiology and
   Biofeedback
10200 West 44th Avenue, Suite 304
Wheat Ridge, CO 80033–2840
(303) 422–8436

Back Pain Association of America
P.O. Box 135
Pasadena, MD 21122
(410) 255–3633
Fax: (410) 255–7338

Biofeedback Certification Institute
   of America
10200 W. 44th Avenue, Suite 304
Wheat Ridge, CO 80033
(303) 420–2902
Web site: www.bcia.org

Fibromyalgia Association
P.O. Box 21988
Columbus, OH 43221–0988
(614) 457–4222
Fax: (614) 457–2729

Fibromyalgia Network
5700 Stockdale Highway, Suite 100
Bakersfield, CA 93309
(805) 631–1950

Help for Incontinent People
P.O. Box 8310
Spartanburg, SC 29305–8310
(864) 579–7900
(800) 252–3337 (BLADDER)

International Chiropractors
   Association (CA)
1110 N. Glebe Road, Suite 1000
Arlington, VA 22201
(703) 528–5000
(800) 423–4690
Web site: www.chiropractic.org

Jaw Joints and Allied
   Musculoskeletal Disorders
   Foundation Inc.
Forsyth's Research Institute
140 Fenway
Boston, MA 02115–3799
(617) 266–2550

Managing Medications
Dept. S
P.O. Box 15329
Stamford, CT 06901
*Send a self-addressed stamped
   envelope for information on
   recognizing adverse drug
   reactions.*

National Arthritis &
Musculoskeletal & Skin Diseases
Information Clearinghouse
One AMS Circle
Bethesda, MD 20892–3675
(301) 495–4484

National Association for Holistic
Aromatherapy
P.O. Box 17622
Boulder, CO 80308
Administrative Office
836 Hanley Industrial Court
St. Louis, MO 63144
(888) ASK–NAHA
(324) 963–2071
Fax: (314) 963–4454

National Chronic Fatigue Syndrome
and Fibromyalgia Association
3521 Broadway, Suite 222
Kansas City, MO 64111
(816) 931–4777

National Commission for the
Certification of Acupuncturists
11 Canal Center Plaza, Suite 300
Alexandria, VA 22314
(703) 548–9004

National Foundation for Depressive
Illness
(800) 239–1263

National Headache Foundation
(800) 843–2256

National Institute of Allergy and
Infectious Diseases
Office of Communications
Bethesda, MD
(301) 496–5717

National Institute of Arthritis and
Musculoskeletal and Skin
Diseases
Office of Scientific and Health
Communications
Bethesda, MD
(301) 496–8188

National Institute of Dental
Research
Information Office
Bethesda, MD
(301) 496–4261

National Institute of Mental Health
Public Inquiries
5600 Fishers Lane, Room 7C–02,
MSC 8030
Bethesda, MD 20892–8030
(301) 496–4000

National Institute of Neurological
Disorders and Stroke
Office of Scientific and Health
Reports
Bethesda, MD
(301) 496–5751

National Medical Association
(NMA)
1012 10th Street NW
Washington, DC 20001
(202) 347–1895

National Mental Health Association
1021 Prince Street
Alexandria, VA 22314–2971
(703) 664–7722
(800) 969–6642

National Osteopathic Foundation
5775G Peachtree-Dunwoody Road,
  Suite 500
Atlanta, Georgia 30342
(770) 452–7100

National Rehabilitation Information
  Center
8455 Colesville Rd., #935
Silver Spring, MD 20910–3319
(800) 346–2742
(301) 588–9284
Fax: (301) 587–1967

North American Spine Society
6300 N. River Rd., #115
Rosemont, IL 60018–4231
(708) 698–1630
Fax: (708) 823–8668

Office of Alternative Medicine
  Clearinghouse
P.O. Box 8218
Silver Spring, MD 20907–8218
(888) 644–6226
TTY/TDY: (888) 644–6226
Fax: (301) 495–4957
Web site: altmed.od.nih.gov

Office of Research on Women's
  Health
National Institutes of Health
Bethesda, MD
(301) 402–1770

TMJ Association, Ltd.
6418 W. Washington Blvd.
Milwaukee, WI 53213
(414) 259–9334

REFERENCES AND
SUPPORTING RESEARCH

"Alternative Medicine: The Facts." *Consumer Reports* (January 1994): 51.

Antonelli, Mary Ann, M.D., and Robert L. Vawter, M.D. "Nonarticular Pain Syndromes." *Nonarticular Disorders* 91 (February 1992): 95–104.

Arthritis Foundation. *Fibromyalgia (Fibrositis),* 1992.

Benson, Herbert, M.D., and Eileen M. Stuart, R.N., M.S. *The Wellness Book.* New York: Birch Lane Press, 1992.

"Bluer Than Blue." *Involved* (Fall 1993): 2.

Clauw, D. J. "Fibromyalgia: More Than Just a Musculoskeletal Disease." *American Family Physician* 52(3) (1995): 843–854.

Croft, Peter, Joanna Schollum, and Alan Silman. "Population Study of Tender Point Counts and Pain as Evidence of Fibromyalgia." *British Medical Journal* 309 (September 1994): 696(4).

Dranov, Paula. "Am I Sick or Am I Tired?" *Ladies Home Journal* 106 (September 1989): 120(4).

Duna, George F., M.D., and William S. Wilke, M.D. "Diagnosis, Etiology and Therapy of Fibromyalgia." *Comprehensive Therapy* 19(2) (1993): 60–63.

"Emotions: How They Affect Your Body." *Discover* (November 1984): 35.

"Exercise: A Little Helps a Lot." *Consumer Reports on Health* (August 1994): 89.

Fauci, A. S., E. Braunwald, K. J. Isselbacher, et al., eds. *Harrison's*

Principles of Internal Medicine. 14th ed. New York: McGraw-Hill, 1997: 1844, 1900, 1955–1956.

Ferguson, Pamela. *The Self-Shiatsu Handbook.* New York: Perigee Books, 1995.

Ferraccioli, George, et al. "EMG-Biofeedback Training in Fibromyalgia Syndrome." *Journal of Rheumatology* 14 (1987): 820–825.

"Fibromyalgia Unrelenting." *The Back Letter* 9 (May 1994): 60–61.

Geel, Stanley E. "The Fibromyalgia Syndrome: Musculoskeletal Pathophysiology." *Seminars in Arthritis and Rheumatism* 23 (April 1994): 347–353.

Griffin, Katherine. "A Whiff of Things to Come." *Health* 6 (November/December 1992): 34.

Hagen, Kathryn. "Feeling Better with Music." *Arthritis Today* 7 (March/April 1993): 19.

Hagglund, K. J., W. E. Deuser, S. P. Buckelew, J. Hewett, and D. R. Kay. "Weather, Beliefs About Weather, and Disease Severity Among Patients with Fibromyalgia." *Arthritis Care Res.* (September 1994): 130–135.

Kjeldsen-Kragh, J., M. Haugen, C. F. Borchgrevink, and O. Forre. "Vegetarian Diet for Patients with Rheumatoid Arthritis." *Clinical Rheumatology* (December 1994): 649.

Kline, Nathan S. *From Sad to Glad.* New York: Ballantine Books, 1974.

Leventhal, L. J., E. G. Boyce, and R. B. Zuerier. "Treatment of Rheumatoid Arthritis with Blackcurrant Seed Oil." *British Journal of Rheumatology* 33 (September 1994): 847–852.

Lipton J. A., R. A. Dionne, eds. "National Institutes of Health Technology Assessment Conference: Management of Temporomandibular Disorders." *Oral Surg., Oral Med., Oral Pathol., Oral Radiol Endod.* 83(1) 1997 (Supplement): 49–183.

Locke, Andrew, M.D., and Nicola Gedees, M.D. *The Woman's Guide to Homeopathy.* New York: St. Martin's Press, 1994.

Lorenzen, I. "Fibromyalgia: A Clinical Challenge." *Journal of Internal Medicine* (1994): 199–203.

Manning F. J., J. A. Barondess, eds. *Changing Health Care Systems and Rheumatic Disease.* Washington, D.C.: National Academy Press, 1996.

McClaflin, Richard R., M.D. "Myofascial Pain Syndrome." *Myofascial Pain Syndrome* 96 (August 1994): 56–73.

McIlwain, Harris, M.D., Debra Fulghum Bruce, Joel Silverfield, M.D., Michael Burnette, M.D., and Bernard Germaine, M.D. *Winning with Back Pain.* New York: John Wiley, 1994.

————. *Winning with Chronic Pain.* New York: Prometheus Books, 1994.

Nathan, Ronald G., Thomas E. Staats, and Paul J. Rosch. *The Doctor's Guide to Instant Stress Relief.* New York: G. P. Putnam, 1987.

Novakoski, Frank, A.T.C. "The Benefits of Weight Training." *Living Well Today* (January 1994): 6.

Nye, David A. "Fibromyalgia: A Guide for Patients." http://www.hsc.missour . . . yalgia/docs/fm-md.html, 1995.

"Optimistic Prognosis for Fibromyalgia Sufferers: Work Disability Uncommon in Decade-Long Study." *The Back Letter* 9 (December 1994): 133(3).

Pillemer, Stanley R., M.D. *The Fibromyalgia Syndrome.* New York: Haworth Press, 1994.

"Probing the Mystery of Fibromyalgia." *Health News* 12 (October 1994): 1.

Selye, H. *Stress Without Distress.* New York: New American Library, 1975.

Sorvino, A. R., E. Kalstrom, and Gene G. Abel. "Biofeedback for Musculoskeletal Pain." *Journal of the American Medical Association* 270(22) (December 8, 1993): 2736(1).

Wartik, Nancy. "Making Sense of Aromatherapy." *American Health* (October 1995): 73–74.

White, Kevin P., Manfred Harth, and Robert W. Teasell. "Work Disability Evaluation and the Fibromyalgia Syndrome." *Seminars in Arthritis and Rheumatism* 24 (June 1995): 371(10).

Wilke, William S. "Treatment of Resistant Fibromyalgia." *Rheumatic Disease Clinics of North America* (February 1995): 247–260.

Wolfe, Frederick, M.D. "When to Diagnose Fibromyalgia." *Rheu-

matic Disease Clinics of North America 20(2) (May 1994): 485–499.

Wurtman, Judith J. "Depression and Weight Gain: The Serotonin Connection." *Journal of Affective Disorders* 29 (1993): 183–192.

Yunus, Muhammad B., M.D. "Fibromyalgia Syndrome: A Need for Uniform Classification." *Journal of Rheumatology* 10 (1983): 841–844.

INDEX